LYME DISEASE

My Search for a Diagnosis

Linda Hanner

Kashan Publishing

P.O. Box 307

Delano. MN 55328

Most scripture quotations are from the King James version of the Bible.

Scripture quotation on page 159 is taken from the New American Standard Bible, copyright, The Lockman Foundation 1960, 1961, 1963, 1971, 1973, 1975, 1977. Used by permission.

Scripture quotations on page 210 are taken from the Revised Standard Version of the Bible, copyright 1946, 1952, 1971, by the Division of Christian Education of the National Council of the Churches of Christ in the USA. Used by permission.

Some names of the people appearing in this book have been changed to maintain the anonymity of persons and events.

Wording of conversations are as close to the actual wording that the author can recall.

LYME DISEASE: My Search for a Diagnosis
© 1991 by Linda Hanner
First softcover printing
(first and second hardcover printings were under the title *Of Power & Love & Sound Mind: Six Years with Undiagnosed Lyme Disease*)

For additional copies write to:
    Kashan Publishing
    P.O. Box 307
    Delano, MN 55328

Printed in the United States of America

All rights reserved.

ISBN 0-9622669-1-4

To my husband, Kim,
and
my four children,
Jerimiah, Jason,
Jennifer, and Jonathan

Acknowledgements

I want to thank the following people who stood by me through my illness and through the writing of this book:

My many friends and family members who believed in me when I stopped believing in myself

Dr. John J. Witek, the most dedicated, caring physician I have ever met

Carol Frick, whose faith in my writing ability and enthusiasm for this project was a great inspiration, and who patiently edited and re-edited so many versions of this manuscript that we both lost count

Jean Perkins, who donated hours of her valuable time helping me rework and smooth out the final manuscript, who helped write the conclusion and prayed this project through to the finish

The many others who offered assistance in a variety of ways

Contents

PREFACE

I first met Linda in early 1985 at a time when she was in the hospital for evaluation of a variety of symptoms. Eventually a diagnosis of Lyme disease was made, but not until three additional years had elapsed, a number of medical specialists were consulted, and extensive and expensive medical testing was undertaken. Ironically, an equivocal result on a relatively simple blood test that had become available led to a possible diagnosis, a course of antibiotic therapy, and gratifyingly, a dramatic resolution of her symptoms. This remission has continued now for almost eighteen months.

In one sense, this is a case report of Lyme disease at a later stage where the physical and neurological symptoms were chronic and intermittent. Being a relatively new infectious disease, only in recent years has the medical community really become aware of it as well as its potential to produce an array of physical and neurological symptoms, and included it in their differential diagnosis. It has gained notoriety as the new "Great Mimicker," joining a list of diseases including systemic lupus erythematosus (SLE), multiple sclerosis, and syphilis among others. Laboratory testing is also quite recent, and at this point the reliability of the serological test and its proper interpretation remain controversial.

From another perspective, this is a document of an individual's and a family's struggle with a seemingly inexplicable problem. It provides testimony to the perseverance of a patient and the resilience of her family which were tested by the series of tribulations that ensued over six years. As a physician, one is accustomed to the limited encounters in an office or hospital room, or over the telephone; the effects of disease and its symptoms on the different facets of a person's life are difficult to comprehend, but in reading this I gained an important awareness.

Finally, this is a generic medical detective story told from the perspective of the patient. It illustrates how elusive a diagnosis can sometimes be. That this is not a new story hints at an important principle relating to the patient-physician relationship. To be effective it requires give-and-take tempered by mutual respect.

Unfortunately, and not uncommonly, a definite diagnosis cannot always be reached. This is often disconcerting for the patient and perplexing for the physician and creates awkwardness in the relationship between the two. When no physical cause can be found physicians need to at least broach the subject of psychological and stress factors, and inquire as to whether this is a possibility.

Linda's case demonstrates the fallibility of medical diagnosis. Examinations and tests can fail to identify a disease that is present, they can mislead (the proverbial "red herrings"), or multiple diseases can simultaneously be present. The interpretation of data from a physical examination and diagnostic tests is partly an art, honed by past experiences. A physician can make an error, can misinterpret, can believe that a certain test result is insignificant. The physician's best protection is an open and critical mind, ready to re-evaluate if future information does not jibe with prior data or conclusions. An active, open patient-physician interaction nurtured by trust and respect, is essential.

The humanness of both doctors and patients becomes apparent in this account. I would hope that Linda's case is reasonably unique and that the majority of the time, after a reasonable period of evaluation, physicians' diagnoses are accurate. Frankly, the acceptance of the medical evaluation process by patient and physicians is predicated on this.

John J. Witek, M.D.
Neurologist

INTRODUCTION

I am writing to tell you about a time in my life—the years between 1981 and 1987—when I was plunged into a physical, emotional, and spiritual battle by an illness that defied medical tests and baffled doctors for six and a half years. During those years I suffered from a bizarre array of symptoms—severe aching, joint pain, weakness, fatigue, night sweats, heart palpitations, uncoordinated gait, impaired speech, chest pain, shortness of breath, numbness and tingling, headache, loss of bladder control, and muscle spasms that jerked my body into unnatural contortions. I consulted twenty-nine physicians and specialists and ingested over twenty different kinds of medication. Dozens of diagnostic tests proved inconclusive for any known illness.

I was brought to a state of such deep despair I became convinced that suicide was my only hope of escape. In a drug-triggered psychotic state, I believed that it was my fate to be forever locked up in some dark place, a prisoner of my own terror, abandoned by God.

My husband vascillated between anger and frustration; trying to protect himself and his feelings from anticipated loss and changes in our relationship and lifestyle, to reaching out to me with love and support. Our children felt powerless and bewildered, yet tried to comfort me in their own tender ways.

Doctors finally discovered that the culprit of my long list of ailments was Lyme disease. Following treatment I recovered dramatically and am once again fully restored to my joyful role as wife and mother and am active in my church and community.

I am deeply grateful to God for my renewed health, but I believe that the true miracle of healing was worked upon my broken spirit before the diagnosis and treatment. My faith in God before my illness had been strong—the corner-stone of my life, I thought. But it shattered in my long struggle with the unknown, the nameless enemy. I cried out to God and heard no answer—or so it seemed at the time. Now, I can look back and see that even in my despair I learned, I grew. God was guiding me through the darkness. Even as I felt my physical condition deteriorating, I came to accept my situation—that my illness was probably unknowable and untreatable. I knew that God was with me. My healed spirit gave me strength and serenity for whatever lay ahead. My prayers had been answered in God's wisdom, and I no longer expected or needed to know the name or to be cured of the physical disease.

That I *was* cured, freed from the disease as suddenly as I'd first been engulfed by it, was an added blessing, further proof of God's grace.

I am compelled to reach out to others who may find themselves or their loved ones in the troubled places where I have been. My book is for those who suffer from Lyme disease, undiagnosed illness, or from depression. It is for those who have become frustrated in their dealings with medical science and the medical profession. It is for those who are struggling with their faith for whatever reason.

Without my faith in God, this book would have been left unwritten. Without Him life would come and go for each of us with all of its pain and problems and there would be no purpose in it. I believe that God alone has the power to give sense, order, and meaning to our lives.

What follows is my story, my journey toward the light. I pray that it will comfort, inspire, help and serve.

1

Summer 1981- Before the illness

I make a right turn and pedal my bike up the stretch of our tarred driveway leading to the storage shed. As I dismount and walk to an empty spot among the assortment of garden equipment and lawn mowers, I can't help feeling a bit smug. As a 33-year-old mother of four, I'm in good physical shape. I was out of bed by six this morning, gave my own house a pretty good once-over, cleaned house for one of my customers, weeded my garden, and mowed a section of our yard. After preparing dinner for the family and tidying up the kitchen, I was still brimming with energy and decided to bike the ten-mile trip with Jerimiah, my oldest son, to his ball practice. The full day has left me feeling invigorated rather than tired.

My bike parked, I sit on the back steps awhile surveying our property. Although it's been over six years since we moved here, I am still a little awed when I think that this house and property belong to us. As soon as the realtor drove us out to look at the big blue century-old farm house we knew it was what we wanted. It appeared massive then in comparison to the small grey crackerbox house we were moving from. Although it needed work, it was a far cry from the other handyman's-dream-homes that we had tromped through in our search for a place that was within our price range and fit our needs.

A distance of land on either side separates us from our neighbors. Only a few miles away from the small town of Delano and a half-hour drive from Minneapolis, we enjoy the peacefulness of country living. Occasionally, when we look out our porch window, we see deer crossing the road and passing through the alfalfa field. They gracefully jump our white picket fence and head back to the park reserve beyond our property.

Kim, my husband, has converted the two-and-a-half car garage into a shop for his cabinet business. Other buildings provide storage for the menagerie of animals he has collected: chickens, ducks, goats, geese and—when we can get them to stick around—a couple of barn cats. He and the children see to it that the animals are fed and watered, the eggs collected and the goats milked twice a day.

The garden is my project. As I look out on it now I reflect on the past. In a sense, that garden was instrumental in leading me to the place I am now in my spiritual life. Every year since we moved here I've planted the 50 by 150-foot patch. I love being outdoors in the warm weather and gardening provides a good excuse. As soon as the last traces of snow melt, I'm armed with shovel, hoe, and seed packets ready to attack the soil. I'm often outside before the children are out of bed. Working to the background of singing birds, I lose myself in thought, prayer, meditation. The warmth of the early morning sun feels good against my skin. A few weeks after planting, I'm eagerly checking for the first signs of green leaves pushing their way through the heavy soil, reaching for the light. I never really expect them to make it and I marvel every time they do. Over and over those tiny plants serve to reinforce my belief that there must be a God, a greater force, far more magnificent than any earthly being. For a long time, though, I wondered whether He ever took notice of me or any of the prayers that I offered. Although I was brought up in a church-going home my convictions were weak. I longed for something to give my life direction and meaning.

After moving here we started attending a small Presbyterian church and, in the spring of 1975, decided to become members. At that time the minister asked us if we believed that Jesus Christ was the son of God and if we had accepted Him as our personal savior. Kim and I both answered yes. Although we never discussed it, I sensed that Kim was more sincere than I in his response. I answered affirmatively only because I didn't know what else to say. I was filled with doubt, unsure what I believed.

It wasn't until almost a year later that I experienced a major turning point in my spiritual life. I was pregnant then and less than excited about it. We had dropped maternity coverage on our insurance and I'd just sold every piece of baby equipment we owned at a garage sale. On a hot summer day like today I went out to the garden to discover that swarms of tiny beetles had invaded it devouring almost every vine and leaf on the plants I'd worked so hard to nurture since early spring. My sense of futility about life in general magnified as I sprawled on my bed exhausted and nauseated from the pregnancy. A line that I had once learned from Shakespeare seemed depressingly real—"Life's but a walking shadow, a poor player that struts and frets his hour upon the stage, and then is heard no more...." That's all I seemed to be doing most of the time—strutting and fretting.

It was then that I finally poured my heart out to God, admitting for the first time in my life that I had no real faith. The only concept I believed for sure was that two forces existed in the world—good and evil. I wanted to be on the good side, whatever that encompassed—the side of harmony and love. I asked the God of Love to show me what He wanted me to believe in, telling Him that I was open to anything whether it be Christianity or some other form of religion. I wasn't sure how He could answer me. I didn't expect a loud booming voice from the sky. I had taken a tremendous risk. If God didn't respond, I would be forced to accept that either He hadn't heard my prayer or that He was unwilling to make himself known.

The following Sunday I was taken aback when an acquaintance came up to me after the service and handed me a book, saying it was a present for me. My recent prayer flashed through my mind, but I immediately brushed it aside. I was afraid to get my hopes up. This had to be coincidental. I read the book with little enthusiasm, taking nearly a month to finish it. I was so unimpressed with it that not even the name stayed with me at first. However, a tiny segment lodged in my consciousness, refusing to fade. Somewhere in that book it said if I invited Jesus Christ into my life and admitted I was a sinner my life would be changed forever. The idea sounded totally illogical. How could saying a few sentences possibly make a major difference? However, I believe that events a few days later triggered something undefinable. I was in my car, ready to leave on a jaunt to the grocery store, when a familiar feeling of hopelessness engulfed me. I decided I had nothing to lose. With great doubt that it could change anything, I leaned my head on the steering wheel and asked Jesus Christ to come into my life, adding something to the effect "Forgive my sins *if* I've committed any." I couldn't think right then of a single significant thing I'd ever done deliberately wrong. All my life I'd been told how good I was and I guess I believed it.

Nothing remarkable happened immediately, but I felt a slight sense of relief—as though I wasn't fighting something anymore. Gradually, over the next days and weeks, I noticed hope had replaced much of my doubt and fear. Something had happened. A seed of faith was planted.

Yet, a couple of things continued to gnaw at me. I couldn't seem to rid myself of some hostile feelings towards certain people in my life. No matter how much I prayed and tried to talk myself out of those negative feelings, it seemed that they were growing further out of proportion rather than diminishing. It bothered me, too, that I couldn't seem to talk about my faith with anyone, even my own children.

In 1978, two years after my conversion experience, I reached what I see as another milestone in my spiritual journey. Strangely, it occured during what the doctors referred to as a clinical depression. In the midst of a 12-day hospital stay some amazing revelations came. It suddenly dawned on me that when I'd asked God into my life, I'd omitted an important step by not admitting I was a sinner, leaving an obstacle between Him and me. In an instant I realized that sin was more than I had understood it to be—it was more than deliberate wrongdoing. My sin was in the resentment and bitterness that I'd carried around for years. As I realized my own need for forgiveness, God's presence became very real to me, and I understood that people in my life whom I'd resented were vulnerable human beings who also needed love and forgiveness rather than my judgement. Any hurt they had caused me was probably no more intentional than the hurt I could now see I may have caused others. So much was revealed—a lifetime of self-pity and self-centeredness dissolved in such a brief moment. When I was able to confess my own sin, I felt totally engulfed in a sense of love and peace. My depression lifted. I had faith and I had forgiveness. I was ready to move on with my life and learn what God had in store.

I talked to Kim about my enlightenment and to my surprise he was accepting and understanding. The incident drew us closer. I had been afraid he wouldn't understand. More and more I was discovering that his faith was there—quieter, less questioning than mine, evidently instilled and grounded in childhood.

We talk more now about everything, including God, and we seldom go to bed at night without counting our blessings. Kim's business is going well. Our four children are beautiful and healthy. Jerimiah, at thirteen, is the most like me when I was growing up. To him, life is a serious business which he approaches cautiously with a deep sensitivity and politeness. Jason, our eleven-year-old politician, is almost a complete opposite of his older brother. He's outgoing and witty and seems to expect life to fall into place for him. Jennifer started life rather cantankerously, but has emerged a sunny dispositioned eight-year-old. She has my conscientiousness and desire to always be creating. Jonathan, at four, is strong-willed and can be a handful at times. Yet, he

Before the illness

has an irresistible charm and a quickness to show affection
that make it easy to overlook his stubbornness.
Our marriage of fourteen years is solid. Kim has his
faults, but they are outweighed by his virtues. He doesn't
pick up after himself and it takes him an average of three
years to finish any household project he starts, but he's a
patient father, a loving husband and he tells me I'm
beautiful even in the morning when I have no make-up and
I'm definitely not. Laughs and hugs are more frequent than
arguments.
Our lives are busier than ever. In our desire to give
something back for all the good things we've been given,
since 1979 we've opened our home to two young male
refugees from Viet Nam. While helping them to adjust to
our culture I also had the opportunity to befriend another
Vietnamese family sponsored by a local church. The wife's
desire to work inspired me to start a housecleaning
business. It's something we can work on together. I can do
the driving and she can earn money without being hindered
by her lack of English skills. I am involved in other church
and community activities as well. Leisure time is scarce, but
I'm usually enjoying life. I'm really looking forward to next
week, I muse. The children will be spending five days at my
sister Kathy's, about an hour's drive away. We take turns
exchanging children every summer. It gives us each time off
and the cousins enjoy playing together. With a few less
bodies about I'll be able to get at some unfinished projects
and have a chance to catch my breath.
Dusk is beginning to settle in and the mosquitoes are finding their way out of hiding and alighting on my arms and
legs. I swat them off and head inside. That's one disadvan-
tage of country living. It seems that we're battling the in-

sects from early spring until late fall. If it's not the mosquitoes, it's flies and gnats. I dust the garden continually for pests, and invariably we pick ticks off ourselves after much time outdoors. I regard the creatures only as a nuisance, not dreaming a tiny insect could be capable of throwing my life into havoc.

2

Late July 1981 - Onset of the illness

I struggle to make my way across the kitchen, but my legs feel strangely uncooperative, as if the signals my brain is trying to send them are no longer understood. Overcome by weakness, I collapse helplessly in the middle of the floor. For a moment I lay still between the island cabinet and the calico wallpaper, staring at the maze of chair legs in front of me. My heart is pounding as the thought forms in my mind, "I've got to call the doctor back."

Working my way toward the chair legs, I pull myself up to reach the wall phone, wondering if Dr. Carson will be in his office. The receptionist detects the anxiety in my voice and within a few minutes the doctor is on the line.

"Hi. What's up?"

"Dr. Carson, I'm afraid there's something more wrong with me than an ordinary virus," I say, my voice trembling. I describe the growing list of crazy symptoms that have plagued me recently—numbness in the side of my face and right leg, intense aching, a constant urge to void, chills and lack of appetite, and now these extreme weak spells.

Dr. Carson interrupts. "Hey, wait a minute! You're giving me too many symptoms. I think maybe it's time to give Dr. Davis a call."

"I don't need a psychiatrist. I'm sick," I stammer.

"Have you got something against Dr. Davis?"

"No, that's not it. It's just that I'm scared. I feel so awful."

"Well, the blood tests we took the other day came back fine." I interpret the firmness I hear in Dr. Carson's voice to mean that he has no desire to discuss the matter further.

For a moment there is an awkward silence, then I mumble a good-bye and hang up the phone, feeling a mixture of anger and confusion.

I hear the back door open and shut and look up to see Jerimiah. "You okay, Mom?" he asks.

"No—I don't know. I guess I'd better go back to bed. I'm not sure if I can make it, though."

Coming to my side, Jerimiah puts his arm around me. He's small for his age, but has a square, sturdy build and does his best to support my 108-pound frame as I make my way back to the bedroom.

The bedding is disheveled and more than ready to be laundered. Shivering, I pull a blanket over my clammy body. Despite the heat and humidity of the Minnesota summer, lately i feel cold much of the time.

Thoughts flood my mind as I try to make sense out of what is happening to me.

It was a week ago on Monday that things began spinning out of control. I felt odd when I woke up that morning.

Onset of the illness

Something wasn't quite right but I couldn't put a finger on it.

Even though Mondays are usually my slump day there was more to it than that. I felt weak, disoriented, slightly dizzy. Simple things like driving the kids to swimming lessons took extreme effort. The next day was no better. A vague feeling of numbness in the left side of my face became more intense, as if I'd been given a shot of Novocain. Cold waves swept through my body. A gnawing, pressuring pain radiated from my lower back.

I managed to drive the children the twenty miles to Kathy's as planned but when I returned home I fell into bed. The whole week was disappointing. The list of projects I hoped to get at remained unstarted. Most of the time I didn't feel sick enough to want to stay down, yet every time I tried to get up I just couldn't seem to function.

The first time I talked to Dr. Carson he suggested that I had some sort of virus, but when the numbness continued he told me that multiple sclerosis, a brain tumor, or a nerve inflammation could be possible culprits and had me come in for some blood tests. Now he suggests this is all a figment of my imagination. My laundry is piling up and the housework goes undone. Just getting meals on the table is a real challenge. My appetite has dwindled to nothing and being around food is nauseating.

* * *

I startle as I hear the sound of an engine slowing down on the county road and tires rolling up the driveway. Kim must be home from work. He'll be hungry after a long day. I started dinner earlier, but left it half-finished. Slowly I stand up, testing my steadiness, wincing with the pain in my back.

Kim meets me in the bedroom doorway, his dark hair sprinkled with sawdust. "Still sick, huh?"

"I feel lousy."

He follows me to the kitchen and watches as I stoop to pull pans from the drawer below the stove. Even that requires monumental effort. I lean against the cupboard for a few seconds before forcing myself to a standing position.

"Why don't you just let someone else fix dinner and go back to bed?"

"They always make such a mess—besides I'm sick of being in bed. Kim, I just don't know what to do," I lament. "I had another weak spell today. I called Dr. Carson again and he told me to call a psychiatrist."

"What?"

"Apparently he thinks all my symptoms are psychological. It doesn't make any sense, though. I couldn't possibly bring on all this myself. All I can think of is that he's labeled me because of that incident I had three years ago. Maybe he was expecting something to happen again."

Kim frowns as he sets the table. He isn't much for housework, but in a pinch he can help a little. He calls the children in to eat when dinner is ready.

We say grace, then as usual everyone is talking at once. I wish they would all be a little quieter. Right now the noise is unsettling and it's a relief when they excuse themselves and scramble back outside so Kim and I can talk again.

"Maybe you've been overdoing it, Linda. You never take any time to relax," Kim says.

"Well, this week I sure haven't overdone it. I've been in bed more than out. And I haven't gotten any better. These

symptoms fluctuate so much. Every time I think I'm starting to feel better, it hits again like a ton of bricks. I just
don't have time to be sick. I need to get back to work. The
Christian Women's Club style show is next week. I have a
board meeting at my house, the kids have already missed
three days of swimming lessons—"

"Why don't you forget about all that stuff! Nothing is
that important. Promise me you'll just spend another week
resting," Kim pleads.

"I guess I don't have much choice," I say glumly.

The next morning I spend making phone calls, cancelling
everything I have on my agenda for the upcoming days,
praying that the additional rest will turn things around for
me.

But as the week progresses, the numbness in my face persists and the pain worsens. By Sunday I'm tossing and turning restlessly in bed. The pain is everywhere now, fierce,
dominating.

Kim has just returned from the morning church service.
As he stands by his dresser pulling his tie from around his
neck he looks at me helplessly. "Linda, I don't know what to
do for you."

"I don't know either. I can't handle this pain anymore.
My back hurts, my knees hurt, everything hurts—and this
numbness—it's so strange—"

Kim walks out of the room and I hear him dialing the kitchen phone. A few minutes later he is back, saying quietly,
"I called Dr. Carson. He'll meet us at the clinic in a half
hour, so why don't you do whatever you need to do to get
ready."

Obediently, I get out of bed and maneuver my way to the
bathroom, grateful that Kim has taken the initiative to call

Dr. Carson. I wouldn't have had the nerve again after my last conversation with him. Maybe he'll listen to Kim.

I glance in the mirror above the bathroom sink. I've been losing weight. My face looks gaunt and pale, but I feel too wretched to care. By the time I finish brushing my teeth and pulling a comb through my limp hair, my meager supply of energy is depleted, and I need Kim's assistance to get to the car.

Once in the examination room of the clinic, Dr. Carson pokes and prods everywhere I complain of pain, humming to himself. If he is annoyed at having his Sunday interrupted, he isn't letting it show. In the years that he's been our family doctor, Kim and I have both grown fond of him. He usually takes time to explain things thoroughly, and we enjoy his touches of humor.

When he's done prodding, he runs his fingers through his hair, pondering the situation. "I still don't find anything amiss on your exam. There is a little too much albumin in the urine, but no infection. There's a chance that this could turn out to be something exotic—"

Kim, standing in the corner of the room, clears his throat. "Do you think that we should get a second opinion, maybe have her checked by an internist?"

"Sure, we can certainly arrange that. She's in enough discomfort that I think I should arrange to have her admitted to the hospital. I'll have an internist look at her tomorrow."

Kim and I drive home to pick up a few essentials, then go to the the regional hospital twenty miles south. After the nurses have me settled in my room between the starched sheets, Kim kisses me good-bye and heads back home. Tests are ordered for the following day.

Onset of the illness

In spite of the prescribed pain medication and sleeping pills, I can't sleep. Sharp, stabbing pains make me clutch my hands to my chest. I don't see how I can tell Dr. Carson about this new addition to my list of symptoms which he already suggests is too long to be believed.

I am awake when Dr. Carson strolls into my room bright and early Monday morning.

"I've arranged for an internist to see you and scheduled you for a kidney x-ray." In a flash he is heading back out the door, saying lightly, "Of course, this could still turn out to be a neurosis."

I ignore his comment, just thankful that he is following up on Kim's suggestion to get another opinion.

White-uniformed nurses and cleaning women bustle in and out of my room. A ghostly patient is being brought down from surgery on a rattling metal cart. She appears about my age. She groans in pain as hospital attendants transfer her from the cart to the empty bed on the other side of the room. There's already a row of cards and flowers lining the nearby window sill.

A handsome young, blond doctor arrives. "Hi, you must be Linda. I'm Dr. Somers. Dr. Carson asked me to look in on you." He pulls the cloth divider between us and my new roommate. "Tell me about yourself," he urges solicitously, sliding a chair up near the side of the bed.

I recount my symptoms of the past three weeks.

"Have you lost any weight?"

"Some—I just can't eat."

"Does your chest hurt?"

"No," I lie, having convinced myself that the chest pain is a result of stress from the whole situation.

Dr. Somers examines me and asks more questions about

my lifestyle before the illness. "Sounds like you keep youself pretty busy when you're feeling well. Do you think that you've been trying to do too much?"

"Maybe, but I had already planned to drop some things—and the past several weeks I haven't done anything but rest."

"Well, I'll be talking to Dr. Carson and he'll get back to you." Then Dr. Somers is gone and I'm alone with my thoughts while my roommate breathes heavily in a sedated sleep.

What was the word Dr. Carson used yesterday? Exotic. This could be something exotic. I try to push anxiety out of my mind and trust that somehow this will all be resolved. I focus my attention on the tiled, dotted ceiling, counting first the squares, then the dots, and recounting.

My roommate wakes from her slumber when the lunch trays are delivered. Her chatting helps to pass the monotony. "Gee, is this all I get? Clear broth and tea? I'm starved!" she fusses.

"If I could trade with you, I would," I reply, surveying the meal under the shiny domed cover. "I don't feel like eating any of this."

The rest of the afternoon my roommate drifts in and out of sleep. A hospital volunteer stops by to deliver a card to me from a church friend. There is an eloquent handwritten note, along with a verse she copied from the Bible. I read and reread it, drawing comfort from the words.

Later my roommate's visitors create a stir of activity in the room until visiting hours are over. When everything quiets down I pray and silently recite every Bible verse that I can think of in order to ease myself through the long, exhausting night that follows.

Onset of the illness

Tuesday morning I jump to the ringing of the phone by my bed. I'm greeted by Dr. Carson's voice. "Hi. I just wanted to let you know that I discussed your situation with Dr. Somers and we feel that we've ruled out every possibility except MS or some other type of neurological disease."

MS...that was what Betty had, the woman I used to work with at the phone company. "Doesn't MS usually go into remission?" I ask.

"Exactly. That's why I don't see any point in treating you for it at this time. The drugs used in treating MS are steroids and can have serious side effects. Dr. Somers did suggest the possibility of having a spinal tap done, but that can occasionally result in nerve damage and in the early stages it's not likely to show anything. I've decided to leave it up to you whether you want to have one done."

In light of Dr. Carson's explanation, I opt not to have a spinal tap, and he agrees to make arrangements for me to be released from the hospital and see him again in a week.

As I hang up the phone, I feel relieved. They must have ruled out a psychological condition also. The thought of having multiple sclerosis isn't terribly alarming even though I know it's a potentially crippling disease. Betty's went into remission shortly after her diagnosis, and years later when I bumped into her in a grocery store, she appeared to be in the pink of health. The best thing to do, I decide, is to go home and wait for my remission.

I can't reach Kim, so I call my mother to let her know what I learned. She takes the news typically calmly. "You know, Aunt Anne had a neurological disease that at one point doctors suspected was MS, too," she reminds me.

When Kim comes late in the afternoon to pick me up, he is solemn and abrupt as he stuffs my robe into a bag and waits for me to get dressed. His patience for doctors and hospitals is limited.

A wall of hot air hits us as we exit the sterile coolness of the hospital and head for his work van, which is parked near the door. At first there is only the sound of the wind rushing through the windows as Kim drives, his eyes hard on the road. Neither of us is sure what to say. He finally pounds the steering wheel with his clenched fist. "Dr. Carson wasn't that sure about this verdict, was he? I just don't think I can handle it if there's really something seriously wrong with you, Linda! You mean too much to me!"

"Kim, even if I do have MS, it might not be that bad. People can have mild cases of serious diseases. Somehow, I know this will all work out. We just need to put it in God's hands." I tell him about my friend at the phone company, hoping to lighten the mood, but he remains sullen the rest of the way home.

We arrive to a houseful of concerned relatives. No one else is taking the news as serenely as my mother. Other reactions are tearful and emotional.

I am exhausted and ready to lie down. Confined once again within the walls of our small bedroom, I study the familiar furniture that fills it. Kim built our maplewood bedroom set while attending vocational school before we were married. It needs a larger room to do it justice. My eyes are drawn to a gold-framed picture of my Great Aunt Anne on the dresser. Uncle Ed had sent it after her death several years ago. As a child I used to write to Aunt Anne thanking her for cards and money she sent on birthdays, but I never had a chance to meet her. I was told that a mysterious tragic illness rendered her helpless and bedridden for many years before her death. She was almost totally paralyzed, unable even to feed herself. My uncle, a banker, tried unsuccessfully to find a doctor who could help her.

I pick up the picture and slide it from its frame. On the back Uncle Ed had written, "A prayer for Aunt Anne is a prayer for anyone with a neurological disease."

I am a little vague about what exactly a neurological disease is; later I learn that it is any disease involving the brain or spinal cord. Maybe I don't have multiple sclerosis. Maybe I have some other neurological disease—whatever Aunt Anne had. I try to imagine what it would be like not to be able to feed myself, brush my own teeth and comb my hair. The thought sends a nauseating chill through me.

The past few days the numbness has been accompanied by the sensation of a rod shoved through the side of my head. What does it mean? The air in the room is thick, oppressive. My pain seemed less intense in the air-conditioned hospital.

As I listen to the sounds in the other room, trying to form words out of the muffled conversation, I can't help wondering how drastically this illness is going to affect our lives.

The night racks my bones, and the
pain that gnaws me takes no rest
Job 30:17 RSV

3

Late August 1981 - More bizarre symptoms

Moisture is streaming down my body from my forehead to my ankles, plastering my nightgown to my skin. As I stir in bed, Kim reaches over and puts his arm around me, then quickly pulls it away. "You're soaking wet!" he exclaims.

"I know. It's sweat. I'm completely drenched. I guess I'm going to have to get up and change." I climb out of bed, fumble in my dresser for a fresh gown and head for the bathroom. I slide my hand over the wall to my left several times trying to locate the light switch until it dawns on me that it's next to the mirror. I recall that yesterday, while trying to get in bed, I missed completely, landing on the floor, because in my mind the bed was positioned in a spot where it hadn't been for over a year. Although I tend to be a little absent-minded, these incidents seem extreme. I wish I could take a shower to get rid of the sick odor but I'm too wobbly. Instead, I dry off with a towel and put on the clean gown.

In the kitchen I find a bottle of aspirin, hoping it'll at least take the edge off the pain. I don't want to disturb Kim again, so I curl up on the couch in the living room. Through the screened window I listen to the steady rhythmic drone of crickets. As the smell of fresh cut grass drifts in, I try unsuccessfully to dwell on something other than the pain, but it refuses to allow me to sleep.

Eventually I hear the ring of Kim's alarm clock. A few minutes later he emerges from the bedroom, rubbing his eyes.

"Did you get any sleep at all last night?" he asks.

"Not much."

"I'm sorry. I wish there was something I could do for you," he says sympathetically. "I'm going to have to hurry. I have a customer meeting me at the shop in a half hour. I'm getting behind and I have two more kitchens coming in today. I'm just going to have a quick cup of coffee." He returns with a steaming mug in hand and sits in the rocking chair near me. "You don't know how hard it is to see you like this. I feel helpless," he says, emphasizing his statement with a sweeping hand gesture.

"It helps just that you're here and that you care."

"But that's not making you better. Linda, I just want you well again!"

Kim finishes his coffee and I feel the familiar roughness of his beard against my cheek as he leans over to kiss me goodbye. "I gotta go. I'll call later."

I lie still for awhile, trying to sleep. It's no use. Maybe if I can get up and do something it will take my mind off the pain. The kitchen sink is filled with dishes from last night's dinner and snacks. I manage to get most of them washed before the children start waking up and coming downstairs.

More bizarre symptoms

Jerimiah, after greeting me good morning, makes a beeline for the pantry and returns with a box of Cheerios. Ever since he was a toddler he's gotten up bright and early and is ready for breakfast the minute he's out of bed. He gulps down two bowls of cereal, then heads outside to do his chores. The goats are bleating in the barnyard, letting him know that they, too, are more than ready for breakfast.

Jason comes down a few minutes later, his blanket draped around his shoulders. Unlike Jerimiah, he's never hungry until he's been awake a few hours. Jenny and Jonathan come last, giving me morning hugs. I am reminded how lucky I am to have my children. They've been especially well-behaved since I returned from the hospital and are putting out their best effort to help me.

I tell Jenny and Jonathan to hurry and get dressed because Uncle Chuck and Aunt Sandy promised to pick them up and take them to the library this morning. They too have been a big help, taking the younger ones for outings to keep them occupied and driving them places they need to go.

A few hours up is about all I can tolerate. The weakness returns, forcing me to spend the rest of the day in bed.

In the afternoon our neighbors, Mike and Debbie, stop by and say they'll be back to make dinner later. Eventually I hear activity in the kitchen. The smell of cooking food drifts into the bedroom making me queasy.

When Mike comes he brings a bouquet of freshly cut flowers. I'm not used to this much attention. Jenny is setting the table in the dining room. I wish I could get up and join them. It seems so unnatural to have other people caring for my family, fixing our meals.

I need to make another trip to bathroom, but when I

stand, I realize I won't make it on my own. I hate this helpless feeling. The one bathroom in our old-fashioned house isn't exactly in a convenient location. In order to get there I need to pass through both the living room and dining room. I wait until I hear chairs being pushed back and dishes cleared from the table, then call Kim to help me. Halfway there I stop in my tracks. Something is wrong. When I try to continue, my right leg stubbornly refuses to coordinate itself with the left, dragging awkwardly. Kim scoops me up and carries me the rest of the way and then back to bed. Debbie and Mike, watching the ordeal, are disconcerted.

"We've got to do something," Mike says. "I'm going to give my brother-in-law, Bob, a call. He's a doctor. Maybe he'll know."

Within a few minutes, Sally, my friend who is a nurse, stops by on her way home from work. There is a flurry of activity and a myriad of suggestions being tossed around. Amidst the chaos, an eerie sensation that flies are crawling all over my body intensifies and I burst into tears.

"Kim, I really think Linda should see a neurologist," Sally advises. "I don't think a GP knows enough about this type of illness."

Kim throws up his hands. "I already tried to make an appointment with one last week and was told they couldn't give us an appointment without a referral from our family doctor!"

Mike is off the phone now and agreeing with Sally. "Bob says that the only way you'll know for sure if you have MS is to have a spinal tap."

It's finally decided that during Monday's appointment I'll talk to Dr. Carson about seeing a neurologist. Over the weekend, when I am strong enough to get up, I occasionally slip back into a normal walking pattern, but more often than not my gait remains unsynchronized.

On Monday Mom and Dad come over with groceries and Dad drives me to my appointment with Dr. Carson. Conversation, other than formalities, has always been awkward between Dad and me, but I know that he loves me and is really worried.

"Linda, I don't understand why this is happening to you. I wish that it could be me instead."

"It'll be okay, Dad. I'm sure Dr. Carson won't take this so lightly now. He's got to do something."

* * *

Dr. Carson taps my knees with a rubber hammer. He has me extend my arms and touch my fingers to my nose and rub my heels down my shins. "Your neurological exam looks fine," he announces.

"But I can't walk right."

"Well, let's see you walk."

He instructs me to walk the length of the corridor outside the exam room. "Hmmm. Obviously your brain isn't sending the right signals to your muscles for some reason. But you still don't have any hard neurological symptoms and I don't think a spinal tap will show anything."

"My family and friends all think that I should be seen by neurologist," I suggest hesitantly, not wanting to be too pushy.

"Well, okay, maybe it's time to check in with one. I'll make some phone calls and see what we can set up."

LYME DISEASE: My Search for a Diagnosis

An appointment is arranged for me to see a Dr. Steele at the hospital the following Monday. A week seems like a long time to wait. At home family members and friends continue to bombard me with suggestions of doctors they think I should see.

4

August 1981 continued - Brain tests

As I sit on the exam table waiting for the neurologist to arrive, I tuck the paper gown carefully around my body, trying to keep it from tearing right down the front. I rub my palms across the crisp paper to dry them. The last time I remember my hands sweating this much was when I had to deliver speeches in junior high school.

The nurse tells me that the doctor is running a little late today and has gone out for a quick sandwich. I wait and gaze around the room which is furnished with two metal and vinyl chairs and a table with metal instruments arranged in an orderly fashion. The tan walls are bare, with no pictures to break the monotony. It's chilly in here and I wish he'd hurry because I feel slightly dizzy. I try to calm my apprehension. *For God hath not given us the spirit of fear; but of power and of love and of a sound mind* (2 Timothy 1:7).

Finally there is a light tap on the door and Dr. Steele

steps into the room, closing the door behind him. A lanky man with a sharp nose and thinning hair, he seats himself in a chair near the exam table, glancing down at the chart he's holding.

"When's the last time you talked to a psychiatrist?"

I stiffen. Dr. Carson must have informed him of my past breakdown. That's fine, but why is it so important to him that it tops his list of questions?

"Three years ago when I went through a depression. I saw a psychiatrist for a brief period of time, but I haven't felt any need to since then."

"Tell me about your symptoms. When did they start?" he urges.

Once again I relate the saga of the past month. Then he performs a more thorough neurological exam than Dr. Carson had done, testing reflexes, coordination, balance and gait.

"Your gait is pretty unusual. While you're getting dressed I'm going to schedule some tests on your brain," Dr. Steele informs me.

"Why are you ordering these tests? Are you looking for a brain tumor?"

"Yes. But if you do have one, it's not one that you're in any immediate danger from," he says matter-of-factly. "It'll take about three weeks to get the test results back. You can make an appointment at the desk to come back then."

As I leave, the nurse hands me a sheet of instructions with times and locations for the tests. Kim, sitting in the waiting room outside the door, looks up questioningly when he sees me.

When I tell him about the impending tests his face drops. I know that he was hoping the neurologist would have some simple explanation for my symptoms. But I'm glad they're doing tests. There must be something wrong with my brain and I want to know what it is. If they find out, maybe something can be done. At least I'll know what I'm dealing with and can somehow begin to structure my life around it.

On Friday morning we return to the hospital for my EEG. Machines and technicians are much less intimidating to me than doctors. They don't make judgments. They just do their job. The technician chats amiably as he pushes the tiny pins into my scalp.

"You seem real relaxed," he comments. "That's good. It should make this go faster."

"Ouch, that one hurt." I feel a warm trickle of blood on my forehead. I remember once seeing a picture in a biology book of a man with wires sprouting from his head, connected to a machine like this. I had shuddered at the thought. Now it's happening to me.

I'm fascinated with the equipment, which monitors what's happening inside my head and records it on a screen. The technician turns on the EEG and studies the screen as I watch his face for any signs of particular interest. "Would you tell me if you see anything unusual?" I ask him.

"Can't do that. It's up to your doctor to interpret the results. Dr. Steele's your doctor, isn't he? You're in good hands."

He places a strobe light in front of my face, telling me to shut my eyes. The bright lights flash rapidly for several minutes, visible through my eyelids like a veiled fireworks display, then click off.

From the hospital, Kim drives me to a neurology clinic where the other tests are going to take place. He drops me off while he goes out for lunch. I was instructed not to eat or drink anything prior to the CAT scan. That isn't a difficult order to follow. My appetite hasn't returned and I can tell I've lost more weight by the way my slacks fit. I have to wear a belt to keep them from drooping.

A nurse leads me down a hallway to a room where I am placed on a table and my head is thrust inside the opening of a monstrous-looking piece of equipment. It sounds like a freight train rushing over my head as a rotating barrel whirs, taking pictures. After one series of images is completed, someone comes with a needle to inject purple dye into my veins for the purpose of creating sharper contrast for a second set. "Let me know if you start feeling funny, or have trouble breathing," the technician says.

An hour later I am brought to another room and more electrodes are attached to my scalp, this time with glue. "We're going to be doing a VER and BAER to check the brain's response to various stimuli," the technician explains.

I am led with draping wires to a room across the hall, where I stare at a television with alternating checkerboard patterns. "Keep your eyes on the screen. Watch the dot in the center and try not to blink." The people here seem as automatic as the machines.

Another piece of equipment produces rapid clicking noises of various intensities in my ears. The machine does all the work and I doze on a leather couch. It feels good. Restful sleep is so rare lately.

When the clicking fades away, a strong-smelling solvent rubbed forcefully into my scalp dissolves the glue that held the electrodes in place. Kim and I leave the complex array of diagnostic equipment behind, wondering if anything has been revealed. If an abnormality is detected will it be treatable? We do not imagine that this is only the beginning of more than six years of expensive tests and endless waiting only to be told repeatedly that no further light has been shed on the true nature of my problems.

In all thy ways acknowledge Him and
He shall direct thy paths
Proverbs 3:6

5

September 1981 - The spinal tap

Ever since multiple sclerosis has been brought up as the possible culprit of my symptoms it seems to have become everyone's common mission to make sure that I rest. Friends and relatives stop by bringing food, offering to help with laundry, housework, and grocery shopping. I'm not sure what I am capable of doing anymore. Every time I attempt even a small task someone is worrying that I'll overdo. Even Van, one of our refugees, will scold me in his broken English if he finds me next to my sewing machine when he comes home from school.

It's comforting, though, to know that so many people care and they have all made the three weeks between visits to Dr. Steele go much more quickly than I anticipated. I've asked Kim to accompany me to listen to the test results.

"Well, all of the tests are back and nothing abnormal has shown up on any of them. So, where does that leave us?" Dr.

Steele is questioning. "Have you been under any stress lately?"

Have I been under any stress lately! The question seems ridiculously inappropriate. For almost two months I have been too ill to function normally, have been in constant pain, have been told that I may have a serious illness, and have gone through several expensive medical tests. How could I not be under stress? He must be referring to the time before my illness.

"No. We have a close family and I have a strong faith. Before this everything in my life was fine," I respond. I think to myself that any stress I'm experiencing is the *result* of my symptoms, not the cause.

"Well, I guess I have to be honest and tell you that I have a tendency to believe your symptoms could be psychological," Dr. Steele continues. "However, you haven't had a spinal tap yet. I guess we really should do one. There's a chance it may show something."

"Dr. Carson told me that they are risky and can cause nerve damage," I interject. "Is that true?"

"If you think you're going to have problems with it, then you probably will," he retorts.

I bristle at his flippant remark but stifle any response.

He reaches into his briefcase, pulling out a manilla envelope which he hands to me. "I'll arrange for the spinal tap. In the meantime I want you to take this home and fill it out. It's a personality test that might be of some help to us. You can mail it back after it's completed."

Kim was silent throughout the interview and stonefaced on the way home. I wish he would say something to let me know what he's thinking. He's been sympathetic and patient beyond expectation the past few months. I know that

The spinal tap

this ordeal has been just as hard, maybe harder, on him than on me—all these doctor visits, never resolving anything. Why is this thing being so elusive? Why can't we ever walk out of a doctor's office with some kind of answer? Eventually something has to show up somewhere, whatever it is that has invaded my body—my brain—and is disrupting our lives. It bothers me that Dr. Steele brought up the psychological possibility again. I know that's not my problem. I can't help feeling that I have been convicted by my past depressive experience.

I can't bear the silence anymore. "Kim, do you think I could be crazy?"

"No, Linda, I don't think so," he says, glancing over at me with a consoling look. "I just don't understand why the tests aren't showing anything. I'm tired of dragging you around for appointments and I'm concerned about this spinal tap."

I'm not worried about the spinal tap. If my mind is capable of making me sick, I reason, then it should be able to prevent reactions, too.

At home that evening I start filling out the 566 questions on the personality test. I am familiar with the MMPI (Minnesota Multiphasic Personality Inventory) from 1978, and as I skim over it, I note that there are a lot of items pertaining to physical symptoms:

I find it hard to keep my mind on a task or job.

I seldom worry about my health.

I have periods of days or weeks where I can't get going.

My sleep is fitful and disturbed.

My head hurts much of the time.

I am in just as good health as most of my friends.

I am losing weight.

LYME DISEASE: My Search for a Diagnosis

I feel weak all over much of the time.
I have numb sensations in various parts of my body.
Dr. Steele instructed me to respond to the statements as they apply to me now. I don't understand how this can accurately portray my personality. I could have responded very differently a few months ago, but the test has no way of knowing that. As far as I know, the test assumes I'm physically healthy, so any physical symptoms will be interpreted as being psychosomatic.

When I complain to Kim he suggests that I just refuse to take it. I'm worried that if I do they'll be even more convinced I'm neurotic or I'll be labeled uncooperative.

I grit my teeth and follow their orders. I take their tests, answering the questions honestly, even though I believe this is of no value. I mail the completed MMPI back knowing full well that I've painted a picture of a complete basket case—a woman who worries about her health, is plagued with numerous aches and pains, stomach problems, bladder difficulties, weight loss, fitful sleep, numbness and weakness. Dr. Carson couldn't have been more right. I have too many symptoms to be believable.

Until this illness I seldom gave my health a second thought, and rarely went to see a doctor. When I did, it was for ordinary things like throat infections and pregnancy check-ups. I've been basically healthy all my life. I haven't been a hypochondriac. This is all turning into such a jumbled mess. I don't understand why it's happening. My faith tells me that God can work something good out of any situation. Past experiences in my life have proven this true. I need to hang on to that belief.

* * *

The spinal tap

On the day of the spinal tap Kim, faithful Kim, is waiting with me in the emergency room for Dr. Steele to arrive. I can't help overhearing a conversation going on behind the room divider. Another doctor is explaining to a woman who has fallen and shattered bones in her ankle that they will have to put in a pin without using anesthetic. I concentrate on praying for her while we wait.

Dr. Steele arrives carrying a long needle. "Kim, I'll just have you step out for a little while. This won't take long. Linda, you can roll over on your side." I follow instructions bracing myself for a painful experience. I'm surprised when there is very little discomfort, only a slight twinge.

"I want you to stay here and lie still for about four hours, then you can go home, but it would probably be a good idea to spend a quiet evening," Dr. Steele says.

I don't know what he expects I'll be doing. He knows I haven't been very active for quite awhile.

Dr. Steele continues. "I'm going to be sending some of the spinal fluid to the Mayo Clinic for evaluation, and that usually takes about a month to get back. Plan to come and see me near the end of October."

A few minutes after he leaves, Kim is back in the room exclaiming, "A month! I can't believe everything takes so long!"

He is restless, but stays with me for the four-hour wait, leaving only once to go for coffee. I know he has plenty of work sitting at the shop, and this is probably the last place he wants to be whiling away his time.

Kim's mom fretted and stewed when she found out I wasn't going to be kept in the hospital overnight. "Everybody I know who's had a spinal tap has had to stay flat on their back for twenty-four hours! It's not right! I don't care what the doctor says, you're staying in bed until tomorrow."

She insists that Kim bring me to her house after leaving the hospital. I'm not in any shape to argue and I don't mind spending the day with her. She has treated me like a daughter ever since Kim and I first met, and she has a gentle, comforting manner.

As evening approaches I'm elated. There is no trace of a headache other than the rod sensation that was there before the spinal tap. I believe I'm home free and anticipate telling Dr. Steele when I next see him that it went without a hitch.

However, my elation is short-lived. On sitting up, a dull ache spreads over my forehead and rapidly intensifies to a sickening level. Oh God, why does this have to happen now, just when I thought things were going so well? The night becomes an interminable ordeal. Every movement of my head exaggerates my misery, yet the accompanying waves of nausea make it impossible to lie still. My stomach convulses with dry heaves. I wrap a pillow around my head trying to stifle the hideous pain and pray that Mary will sleep through my thrashing.

Early in the morning, after hearing Mary's husband, Bob, bid her good-bye and leave for work, I stagger out to the kitchen and roll down on the floor. "I can't stand this anymore! The pain is excruciating. Please call Kim and ask him to take me back to the hospital. They've got to do something!"

We were instructed to call Dr. Carson if there were any problems, so Mary telephones him first and conveys his instructions. "The doctor said that you must have a spinal leak, and the best thing to do is to stay flat on your back for another twenty-four hours. He prescribed some medication for the nausea," she says, covering me with a blanket and tucking a pillow gently under my head. "Try not to move."

The medication does help settle the nausea down to a more tolerable level, and I manage to keep Tylenol down, but the suffering continues to border on the unbearable.

Two long days pass, then three. Mary patiently attempts to feed me her cure-all homemade chicken soup. "Linda, you've got to eat. You're wasting away!" she coaxes. "Why don't I call Kim and ask him to bring Jonathan here? Then at least you won't have to worry about him. He can miss a few days of nursery school and he'll feel better if he can be with you."

The three older children have been foraging for themselves at home and getting themselves off to school in the morning. Jerimiah has been assuming the role of supervisor and Kim reports that the essentials are being accomplished. I wonder how Jenny is managing to fix her hair. She has sent notes saying "I miss you" and "Please get well" along with pictures she has drawn of butterflies, hearts and rainbows. Jonathan has been juggled back and forth among friends and relatives and does seem glad to see me when Kim brings him.

One afternoon Mary reads a verse from her Bible in her deep, slow, soothing voice. "Is any sick among you? Let him call for the elders of the church; and let them pray over him, anointing him with oil in the name of the Lord" (James 5:14). It's the first time I've ever known Mary to read aloud from her Bible. A little later, the minister of her church stops by and prays for me before leaving. Many others have been praying as well. If I could only get better for them, if not for me.

* * *

LYME DISEASE: My Search for a Diagnosis

A week has gone by and still my headache isn't abating. I can't bear to sit up and my treks to the bathroom take every ounce of stamina I have. I'm beginning to feel like a burden on Bob and Mary. I know her health isn't the best and I worry about her worrying about me! I beg Kim to bring me home, and reluctantly he agrees. Getting out to his van is a major ordeal and I ride sprawled on the floor, fighting back the nausea aggravated by the motion. The slightest bump sends piercing pangs through my skull.

At home I spend the days on the couch in the living room. Kim has placed the phone where I can reach it without getting up. Jonathan has changed from a typically spunky four-year-old to a much more serious, subdued child, hovering protectively nearby. A few months ago I would have had to tie him down to get him to stay this still and play quietly this long. To help occupy him I manage to play board games by positioning my head near the edge of the couch and dangling my arm over the side. He is becoming adept at making peanut butter sandwiches when he gets hungry and even cleans up the kitchen afterward. My caretaker, too, he brings me the mail every day. There are almost always notes with words of encouragement. God seems to be whispering through them that He is still here, that he cares. One card I receive contains the same verse Mary read from her Bible. "Call the elders of the church and let them pray..." We have elders in our small Presbyterian church, but I don't know of any who are in the habit of praying over sick people. I do know of one couple who have mentioned it from time to time. They are newer members and we've become good friends.

It's been a full two weeks now since the spinal tap and my head pain hasn't eased; instead it has spread to include the back of my head and neck. Once more I telephone Dr. Car-

- 42 -

The spinal tap

son. He says it should be better by now and offers no solution. I'm beginning to feel like I'm going to be in this agony for the rest of my life. My sense of foolishness about calling Brian and inquiring about the praying—the oil—is overridden by my desperation to try anything to make life tolerable again. I'm relieved to hear his warm, sincere voice on the line. "We were just on our way to our friend's house. We'll come over in about twenty minutes," he tells me. Good. They'll be here before it's time for the gang to get home from school.

Brian and Jan arrive with their friend, who has a small bottle of oil in hand. All three kneel on the floor next to the couch and lay their hands on me, praying earnestly. As they do, a warm sensation flows through my body. I feel the tension drain, my muscles loosen and my entire body relax.

Soon I hear the children's footsteps on the stairs as they go up to their rooms. When the prayer trio is ready to leave, I still have the headache, but it seems more tolerable. Later in the evening Mom and Dad bring supper and I am able to eat. The next day brings a major triumph when I discover that I can bend over to tie Jonathan's shoes before he goes to nursery school.

Each day I notice further improvement. On Sunday I attend church for the first time since July. I enter the door walking clumsily, my right leg dragging, but it's great to be back. The ushers welcome me with grins and hugs. It was the friendliness of the congregation that had drawn us to join this church originally. I'd been impressed by their willingness to give so much of themselves, quietly, without asking anything in return.

As the organ prelude fills the sanctuary, I feel immensely thankful for these church friends. Kim and I have both felt overwhelmed by the love and support we've received from them during the past months—meals, flowers, driving the children around and prayers. Through so many of them my faith has been uplifted and strengthened.

6

October 1981 - Am I crazy?

It was Kim's idea to take a drive south to Red Wing on this glorious sunny autumn day. It's rare for him to volunteer to take a whole day off work, even on a weekend. The trees we pass are arrayed in a splendor of gold, orange, and deep red. It feels good to be out of the house and heading somewhere other than to a doctor appointment. When Kim spots a park with playground equipment he decides to stop and let the kids work off some of their energy.

Early in July I visited this town with our church youth group on an excursion to climb the Red Wing bluffs. Jonathan tired of climbing half-way to the top, so I finished the trek carrying him, resting him on one hip, grabbing branches jutting from the steep hillside with my free arm to pull the weight of our bodies upward. From the top of the bluff we gazed down at a breathtaking view encompassing miles of treetops and minature roads and buildings. After catching our breath we made our way back down to picnic, swim and play volleyball until we were too exhausted to move.

Now, as I plunk myself on a picnic bench to watch the children, I am just thankful for the strength to be outside enjoying their energy. It's good to see them laugh and play together, their blond heads bobbing as they run. They all have more of the Hanner features, the big eyes and long eyelashes, but lately people are commenting that they see more of me in Jenny. I know the past months have been disturbing them. Jenny's school teacher commented that she's expressed concern about what is happening to me and seems quieter than usual in the classroom. Jason's teacher informed me that one day she spotted him with a book mark with the inscription, "God is greater than any problem I have." When she asked if he believed that, he told her he did. We don't talk about my illness much at home. It's hard to know what to say when we have no definite answers. Yet, overall, they seem to be adjusting well, accepting the fact that I just can't do many of the things I've done in the past. One thing these months have made me painfully aware of is how vulnerable we all are. I pray that these children of ours will always stay healthy.

* * *

A few weeks later, as we drive the winding roads back to the hospital, I notice that the leaves have already lost most of their radiant color and are fluttering to the ground. I know that Kim has the same reservations about this trip that I do. Will we leave knowing any more than we did before we came? It's a catch-22. If something shows on the

Am I crazy?

spinal tap, it most likely won't be good news. If nothing shows, we'll be back to square one with still no answers. When we are once again in the familiar hospital room waiting for Dr. Steele to fill us in, it seems like everything is moving in slow motion. He seems to be talking deliberately slowly, pausing too long. He asks how I fared after the spinal tap and I mention I had a headache, but play down the severity.

"Everything on your spinal looked good... However, your MMPI wasn't normal. It showed you to have a hysterical personality—the type that would be likely to come up with a neurosis," he says, almost hesitantly.

I want to proclaim that I knew the test would come out that way, to try to explain why I don't believe it can be of value, but I remain silent once again.

Dr. Steele goes on. "Of course there's always a chance that the tests have missed something. No test is infallible. A while back a woman came to see me after going through testing at the Mayo Clinic. They found nothing wrong and told her the problem was psychological. Six months later I repeated the tests and discovered a brain tumor... So I guess we can't rule out the possibility of a brain tumor. Or in your case, MS. I could refer you to another neurologist if you want, but most people who go from one doctor to another are hypochondriacs. I could be wrong, but taking everything into consideration, I still have strong inclinations to believe your symptoms are psychological. I would suggest that you see a psychiatrist, but it's really up to you. Otherwise you could come back in six months and we can re-evaluate you're situation."

I sit expressionless, stifling the anger, fear, and dismay that are welling up, making me feel like I'm going to explode from the pressure. Inside my thoughts are racing, yet I manage to respond evenly, "Okay, I'll make an appointment with the psychiatrist."

A few minutes later as Kim pulls our car out of the parking lot, hot tears spill over my cheeks progressing to uncontrollable sobs. He looks at me in astonishment. "I don't believe it! You appeared so calm in there!"

"I know," I blurt. "I felt I had too! If I show that I'm upset, it'll just further convince them that I'm hysterical. I'm so tired of being sick and not knowing why! Dr. Steele seemed so sure of himself. I know all these symptoms can't be in my head. He said there is a chance he is wrong and he *is* wrong. I'm not hysterical, I'm not crazy!" Yet, even as I declare my belief in my mental soundness, doubts are creeping in. With so many symptoms, at least one test should have picked up a clue. Oh God, I'm not sure of anything anymore.

"It'll be all right, honey. We'll figure out something." He tries to sound reassuring, but I detect uncertainty and exasperation in Kim's voice, too. He pulls off the road near a park bench. We sit for what seems an eternity in the cool autumn air, the silence broken only by my sniffling and the stirring of the dried leaves being gently tossed by a slight breeze. The green paint on the bench is chipped and peeling. I pick off a chunk, crushing it between my fingers, watching it flutter toward the ground. I have an awful feeling, like I too am being crushed, body and soul, and falling helplessly into an evermore frightening unknown.

When I finally regain my composure we climb back into the car and head home. There's nothing more we can do now except wait some more, wondering if I have multiple sclerosis, a brain tumor, or am simply crazy.

7

Late October 1981 - Reactions

At first I'm reluctant to tell my family and friends that Dr. Steele seems convinced that my illness is psychological. I'm not sure how they'll respond. Maybe they'll believe that I've put them through all this worry and concern for nothing and be angry. I fight feelings of guilt. I can only think of two reasons to come up with a psychosomatic illness—as an attention getter or as a self-punishment. Have I been enjoying all the attention this illness has created? It doesn't fit. I have too many things going for me. I feel loved and noticed. I don't feel I deserve to be sick. I'm in a constant paradox. If I push myself to try and do things, my family and friends are anxious I'll make my condition worse. Yet the doctors say there's no reason I shouldn't be functioning normally, and if I stay inactive they will imply that I'm pampering myself.

Maybe the doctors are right. After all, I'd probably be the

last person to know if I were emotionally disturbed.

I talk to myself. "There's nothing wrong with you, Linda. Forget about the illness. Maybe you're over-reacting. There's no reason you can't do the things that you've always done. The housework shouldn't be such a big problem. You used to breeze through the whole thing in a couple of hours. The place really needs dusting. That should be easy enough. There, you did two end tables, the piano, the TV cabinet! Just keep moving. The dining room comes next. And the kitchen is a disaster. It always feels good to get that done."

But it's no use. I'm wiped out. I can't do any more. I kneel on the carpeted floor by the coffee table and bury my head in my arms. Maybe I should call Dr. Steele back and tell him to go ahead and admit me to the psychiatric ward. I don't have the strength to fight this anymore. I'm weary of the raging pain keeping me awake most of the night, of the endless trips to the bathroom, of this distracting rod wedged through the side of my head, of racking my brain to try and figure out why on earth I would want to feel so rotten. Dear God, I wish someone would just tell me what to do. I'm too tired, too weak, and I hurt too much to make any decisions.

Babe, our dog, is barking. Someone is knocking at the door. Get a grip on yourself and go answer it. It's Carol, sweet thoughtful Carol, a friend from church. "Hi, I had to come over this way, so just thought I'd stop and check up on you to see how things are going."

"Thanks. I'm doing okay," I lie.

I invite her in for a cup of coffee and we sit down at the kitchen table. I realize from the look of concern in her soft green eyes that she's seeing through me. "Are you sure you're all right? You don't look real good."

Reactions

"Carol, my doctor doesn't think there's anything physically wrong with me. Nothing showed up on the spinal tap. He recommended a psychiatrist. Maybe that *is* what I need." I quickly look down at the table, biting my quivering lip.

Carol reaches across the table and grabs both my hands, holding them firmly. "Linda, look at me! I don't believe for one minute that this is in your head, nor is there a single person in our church who does. There is something physically wrong with you! The doctors just haven't found it yet. You're not the type of person to come up with a fake illness. You're not a complainer."

"Oh Carol! I'm so confused. I don't know what to do."

"Well, I want you to know that we're all a hundred percent behind you. Don't give up! There's got to be a doctor somewhere out there who can help you."

Almost everyone I know responds with the same kind of indignation as Carol. Some even offer to sign petitions and bring them to the doctor's office stating their belief that I am not a hypochondriac. At times it amazes me that they believe so strongly in my mental soundness, in spite of the fact they all know I've had a breakdown in the past.

Only one friend, out of all of them, suggests that my illness might be psychosomatic. I lash out at her angrily only to regret it afterward. After all, what do I expect? I have my own doubts. I call her back and apologize. But she stops calling me after that. Before, we talked often and our children played together. The absence of her friendship leaves an emptiness. I call her now and then, but the conversation is always strained. I didn't mean to hurt her. I just want my life to be back to normal.

The days all blend together. Kim and I used to get together with friends on weekends. I miss the socializing. Kim seems more content than I am just to stay home. He worries about me having problems when we're out. Some days are better than others and there are times when I can walk almost normally. On those days I convince myself that I've at least been blowing things out of proportion. But when the symptoms worsen again, I know I'm not exaggerating. I can think of a million better ways to get attention.

Days are bearable, but during the night, when the pain gnaws mercilessly through my body, I lie in bed analyzing the situation to death. I've gone over my breakdown a thousand times comparing every detail, every feeling to what I'm experiencing now. Back then I'd been tense, resenting an overload of demands I felt were being placed on me. I just wanted to run away from it all. There had been no associated physical symptoms and I never tried to deny that the problem was mental. I hadn't balked at seeing a psychiatrist. My current illness is different. I wasn't feeling depressed or out of control before my symptoms came on. And now I don't feel like running away from anything except this unrelenting pain. I feel no significant resentment toward anyone in my life. All my prayers and soul searching continue to bring me to the conclusion that some cruel destructive organism has contaminated my body, but for some reason it's defying the medical tests.

8

November 1981 - Groping for answers

I told Dr. Steele that I'd make an appointment with the psychiatrist, Dr. Davis, and I follow through hoping to get some professional affirmation of my mental soundness. Surely he'll be able to see that I'm mentally okay and maybe he can convince Dr. Steele that the answer to my problem isn't psychiatric care.

Dr. Davis was assigned to my case three years ago when I was hospitalized for the breakdown. I never got to know him very well then. At first I'd been too weepy to talk and was in such a confused state I couldn't even remember what time to go for meals. A week afterward I'd announced confidently that I was ready to go home and that I wanted to discontinue my medication. Dr. Davis had been understandably skeptical. He even tried to talk me into staying longer. My healing from the clinical depression was dramatic —probably too dramatic to be accepted by the psychiatric staff.

LYME DISEASE: My Search for a Diagnosis

Back then I had cancelled a scheduled follow-up appointment with Dr. Davis following my recovery and release from the hospital. Part of me had wanted to go, just because I thought it would be interesting to talk to him about the incident and the spiritual healing and new perspectives I received at that time. Yet I couldn't justify spending scarce money on the appointment when I felt that I was functioning and feeling well.

The impression I'd retained of Dr. Davis was neutral. He was just a doctor who had been there, so he seemed the logical one to talk to now.

He sits tilted back in his chair behind his desk, folded hands pressed against his dimpled chin. I shift from one side of my chair to the other, feeling a little uneasy under his penetrating gaze. He listens intently for forty-five minutes, occasionally interjecting a question, as I recite the events of three years since I last talked to him.

Toward the end of the session after a quick glance at his watch he says, "Linda, I have no way of knowing whether your symptoms are real or psychological. We could start you on some antidepressants and just see if they help."

I remind him that when I was put on antidepressants before, I had trouble with my blood pressure dropping so low that I blacked out. He says I'd have to stay in the hospital to be monitored.

I decline his offer and as I get up to leave, Dr. Davis follows me to the door patting me lightly on the shoulder. "I really think that your back pain and bladder problems might be caused by sexual frustrations."

I can't believe that I've spend eighty dollars to have him tell me that! Now I *am* getting depressed.

People continue to offer advice. Brian and Jan encourage

me to see the chiropractor who helped Brian's daughter with some unusual problems. I go because they're good friends and I respect their advice and because my symptoms are so unrelenting, even though I'm not convinced a chiropractor can help.

The chiropractor draws blood and cuts hair samples from the nape of my neck, has them tested and later informs me that I am low on several vitamins and minerals. I figure the tests must have some validity because my insurance pays a portion of them. I buy the vitamins that he recommends, all seventy-five dollars worth. It's peanuts compared to what we've already spent on medical bills. I'm willing to try anything now, and vitamins seem to make sense. I begin reading books on nutrition. I haven't been eating right since I've been ill, and even before that I often skipped meals when I was busy. Maybe poor diet has contributed to or is aggravating the situation.

A friend brought me a locally-produced concoction and touted cure-all consisting of hydrogen peroxide and water. It burns my throat and leaves an awful taste in my mouth, but I drink it, in case there is a chance this remedy will help. She is convinced that it has put her cancer in remission.

I see a gynecologist and he performs exploratory surgery, but can't find the source of the searing pain in my lower pelvic area. I ask to see a urologist because I really think it's got to be inside my bladder, but my requests for a referral are ignored.

Kim's family is convinced I should go the world-famous Mayo Clinic in Rochester. However, Dr. Steele has said the equipment available there is no more sophisticated than what he has available to him, and the thought of going through more tests and not finding answers is too disheartening. Besides, I've heard it takes about five days to be evaluated at the Mayo and Kim just can't afford to take that much time off work to take me. He's already missed too much on my account.

Normally I'm not a reader, but now I read books—medical books, books on healing, and more books on nutrition. I look up every verse in the Bible on healing and read them over and over again, memorizing some, claiming the promises they offer.

I do my best to live with this from day to day. My life has changed so much. I used to feel like I'd wasted half my day if I wasn't out of bed by six in the morning. Five-thirty was better. Then I really felt on top of things. Now I often sleep until nine because my nights are so disrupted by pain. I no longer see Kim off to work and if I'm still in bed the kids quietly ready themselves for school without disturbing me. I no longer work and I'm not involved in church, school or community activities. I fight emotional distress as well as the physical symptoms. Feelings of guilt and worthlessness accompany me. I am more the patient than the wife, mother, and friend I want to be.

9

Late November 1981 - More doctors

I pick up the phone wondering if it's Kim calling me from work. He calls every day to check on me. His concern is reassuring. Before the illness I never heard from him during work hours.

"Hi, hon. Guess what? Remember that Dr. Isaacs, the neurologist we saw on the news last night—the one who specializes in MS?" I do remember him—he talked about the difficulty in diagnosing the disease. Kim sounds uncharacteristically excited. "Well, I called his office today and got an appointment for you to see him on December first!"

I didn't think neurologists would see new patients without a referral, but Kim says they didn't hesitate to set up an appointment when he explained my situation to them.

I'm starting to let myself hope again. Maybe this doctor will at least be able to tell me how likely multiple sclerosis is in my case. And maybe it'll be good to see a doctor who hasn't been briefed on my history beforehand. He'll be able to form his own opinion.

December arrives with moderate temperatures and only light snowfall. Every day I've been faithfully taking the vitamins the chiropractor prescribed. My symptoms aren't going away, but I've been eating better and feeling stronger. On the way to my appointment with Dr. Isaacs Kim and I are optimistic. As I gaze at the winter landscape my thoughts go to a pamphlet Mom brought me from the library a while back. It was about multiple sclerosis and it describes almost every symptom I have except for the pain. The pamphlet also says that the disease is extremely difficult to diagnose in some cases, that it can take as long as five years. Kim reaches over and grips my hand tightly. "I'm praying that this guy has some answers for us," he says.

On arrival Kim and I are ushered into an examination room where a young dark-haired nurse interviews me for background information. Dr. Isaacs enters and chats with Kim for a few minutes, asking about his business and making small talk. He's a slight man with a quick energetic manner. I'm relieved that he seems friendly.

As the doctor conducts the neurological exam, I feel I could go through the paces without prompting, it's becoming so familiar. When he asks me to stand with my feet together and eyes closed, I am unable to without falling to one side. I've noticed lately that my balance seems off. Getting up at night to go to the bathroom, I veer to the right and bump into the wall.

"Step outside and walk down the hall for me," he instructs.

More doctors

As I walk the length of the corridor and back again, my right foot turns inward, my toes drag across the carpeting. My month-old shoes have a spot near the toe-end where the continual dragging has almost worn a hole through the leather. Dr. Isaacs squats to study my unusual gait, rubbing his chin. Back in the exam room he seems to be thinking aloud. "A brain tumor could cause you to walk that way... But it couldn't cause that whole array of symptoms."

Then, looking at both Kim and me, he begins to explain. "We have four categories we can put people into when considering MS. We classify it as definite MS, probable MS, possible MS, or definitely not MS. I would have to classify you as possible MS." He seems to ponder the situation a moment longer and then adds, "One thing we could do for you is admit you to the hospital and try some cortisone injections to see if they help."

"Is that what you're recommending?" I ask.

"Not necessarily. It's just one possibility."

I hesitate, recalling that our family doctor said cortisone is a steroid and can sometimes be dangerous. Then I tell him about the vitamins I've been taking. "Since I started taking them I seem to be doing a little better. Do you think it would hurt just to keep taking them for now and see if things continue to improve?"

Dr. Isaacs doesn't think they'll be of much value, but tells me to go ahead and try them if I want to, since they probably can't hurt.

Having received Dr. Isaacs' initial evaluation I'm ready to share my psychiatric background. He and Dr. Steele both work out of the same clinic and he'll probably see it in my medical records anyway. I begin, "Dr. Steele has suggested that my symptoms might be the result of a neurosis. I did have one depressive episode in the past, but never any symptoms like these before."

As soon as I speak I sense a change in Dr. Isaacs. "Oh?" His voice is suddenly abrupt. "I'll see you again in one month. But before our next visit I want you to set up an appointment with a psychologist who works with some of my patients. Talk to the receptionist at the desk and she'll set it up."

Kim is not happy about this. On the way home he stews, "I don't like the idea of you going to the psychologist. Haven't you gone through enough of that? You were upset for three days after seeing Dr. Davis." But I've already made the appointment and I decide I'll go since that's what Dr. Isaacs wants.

I keep taking the vitamins and am feeling some improvement. I'm still far from well, but I manage to keep the housework from getting too far out of hand by tackling just a little at a time and resting a lot. Friends and relatives are still offering help, but I don't need to rely on them as much. I want so much to feel productive again. I used to have my next day planned before I went to bed at night and went strong till the end of the day. Now I'm grateful for any accomplishment, no matter how small.

10

Winter 1982 - The new year

Somehow we got through Christmas. Kim took a more active role than usual, shopping for gifts for the children. An, our older refugee, moved out earlier in the fall. Van is still with us and since he has obtained his drivers license he can run errands for me. On Christmas Eve and Christmas Day the relatives came to our house and took over most of the food preparation and clean-up.

After four months of not driving, I've begun venturing out on my own more. Even though my right leg and foot aren't coordinated when I walk, I can control my foot well enough to drive. My appointment with the psychologist is today and I feel confident enough to drive myself to her suburban office. She will be the fifth doctor I've seen from this same clinic.

Dr. Banes, a fair, medium-built woman with a businesslike manner, has no idea why I've come to see her. I would have thought Dr. Isaacs would have briefed her when he made the referral, at least sent her some records. I start from the beginning to describe the past six months, then I explain about my past depression and the time between that and my illness. As I talk I begin to feel relaxed. It's easier for me to open up to her than some of the other doctors who seem so sure of themselves, raising their eyebrows at any suggestion that isn't their own.

I explain to her that I wasn't feeling out of control when these current symptoms started. I tell her about the results of the MMPI that Dr. Steele requested.

"The MMPI isn't really accurate in a situation like yours," she comments. "There are other psychological tests that would be better."

I can't believe it! She is echoing the very thoughts I had while taking the test. And she is a professional, someone who should know. She continues, "From talking to you I don't get the feeling that you have serious emotional problems. You seem to have a pretty good handle on your situation. I can do some further testing just to make sure though."

She leaves the room and returns with a copy of the Rorschach test. I remember taking it in 1978. Then, I had stared vacantly at cards of ink blotches as the tester had impatiently tried to get me to describe what I saw in them. I hadn't been able to recognize anything familiar. But now as Dr. Banes proceeds, I identify in the ink spots shapes of birds, bats, butterflies, kidneys, seahorses, flowers, people...

When I return to her office a few days later she has evaluated the results. "I compared your testing to those you took before and it shows much improvement. In fact there is no indication of anything abnormal including depression. I can tell you some things about your personality—you're a caring person, somewhat of a perfectionist, you tend to take on a little more than you can handle at times, and it bothers you when things aren't organized. However, you don't appear to me to be the kind of person likely to come up with a psychological illness nor does the testing indicate that you are. I can't tell you whether or not your symptoms are caused by MS. But I can tell you that your difficulty in getting a diagnosis and your frustration is typical of those who have it."

I am thrilled with her verdict. "Can you send copies of your evaluation to my other doctors?" I ask.

"Sure. Just write down the names and addresses for me, and I'll see that Dr. Isaacs reveiws them, too. I guess there's no reason for you to come back to see me again. I wish you luck, Linda."

I can't believe that I'm actually leaving a doctor's office feeling like something has been resolved! I've made progress. An expert has pronounced me mentally normal. Now maybe the doctors will at least rule out that possibility. I stop at Kim's office on the way home and we go out for lunch to celebrate.

However, after my meeting with the psychologist I am disappointed that Dr. Isaacs makes no mention of ever receiving a copy of Dr. Banes' evaluation or talking to her. I thought that, because he suggested I see her, he would value her opinion. Instead, he is more curt than ever. When I complain that my balance is so far off that I can't close my eyes to pray in church he quips, "Well, don't close your eyes then!" When I complain about the constant nerve-wracking pain and pressure in my bladder he sighs, "Okay, I'll refer you to a urologist, but only as a one-time thing." I think to myself that maybe it is too much to expect him to give me answers when he has none to give.

Later I obtain copies of my records. In them he has written, "This patient insists on an organic explanation for everything, including her bladder symptoms. I feel there is none."

By February my head sensations are almost driving me to distraction. Because the rod is on the left side of my head, and my right leg is the affected one, I wonder if there is some correlation between the two. I've read that the left side of the brain controls the right side of the body. When I tell Dr. Isaacs that it feels like there is something lodged in my head that doesn't belong there, he tells me I'm hyperventilating. I disagree. I never experience any gasping for breath or light-headedness that I understand to be connected with hyperventilation. The rod never leaves; I don't see how I can be hyperventilating constantly. But when I question it he retorts, "What do you want me to do, cut your head open?" He sends me home with a prescription for tranquilizers, tells me to breathe into a paper bag and to start walking two to three miles a day.

As we drive home from that visit the tension is almost palpable. I sense that Kim is reaching the end of his rope. He's been so good about all of this. How will I ever make up to him and everyone else all the trouble I've put them through? I look out on a gloomy, overcast February day, a perfect match for my drooping spirits.

"The guy's a jerk," Kim mutters half to himself.

After he took the time and trouble to arrange our meeting with Dr. Isaacs, hoping to come closer to an answer, our encounters have only added more weight to our distress. A tight knot is forming in the pit of my stomach.

The new year

At home Kim flops on our bed and falls asleep, too tired and depressed to go back to work. He just wants to shut everything out. This illness is taking its toll on all of us. While he dozes I go outside in the dreary, misty cold and force myself to walk along the shoulder of the county road, edged with gritty half-melted snow and ice. I am determined to follow the doctors' orders. I'll walk; I'll breath into a paper bag twenty-four hours a day if it'll do any good!

I return from the excursion exhausted, swordlike pains jabbing through my chest with every breath. My head feels split in two. Breathing into a paper sack doesn't help relieve the head sensations. I keep trying to walk during the next few days, but finally decide to listen to my own screaming instincts that are telling me I'm too sick. I save what energy I have to care for my family.

*For I reckon that the sufferings
of this present time not worthy
to be compared with the glory which
shall be revealed to us*
Romans 8:18

11

Fall 1982 - Grasping at straws

It's past time to get up and I feel like I'm drowning in a sea of pain. It doesn't do any good to lie here and dwell on it. Time for the morning pep talk. Remember, it's usually better after you're moving. Your head will feel better, too. If you keep busy you won't notice it as much. I kneel by my bed and repeat my ritual prayer. "Dear God, I don't know what's wrong with me, the doctors don't know, but You know. Help me to keep this in Your hands."

A few days earlier, when I was having an especially bad day, I opened my Bible and the first verse I read was in Corinthians. *For our light affliction, which is but for a moment, worketh for us a far more exceeding and eternal weight of glory* (2 Corinthians 4:17). I felt uplifted by that verse and I've memorized it. It is my sign from God that He's still with me.

This world is temporary, my life is temporary, therefore

this illness is temporary. There will be better things beyond this if I can just get through it.

This illness hasn't been all bad. At least it's forced me to slow down. I'm taking time to do things I seldom did before—writing letters, reading, joining a Bible study group—things I was usually in too big a hurry for. I'm more patient now in helping the children with their homework and other more sedentary things. I've always found it easier to do all the housework myself. Out of necessity the children have been taking on more responsibilities, and I'm learning to let some projects go.

If I pace myself, I get through most days pretty well. Some are better than others. I never feel healthy—at best it's as though I'm constantly on the verge of the flu, chilled and feverish, but the pain is usually manageable. Maybe I've learned to cope better, to relax instead of tensing up. Perhaps things have leveled off and won't get any worse.

It's been almost a year since the onset of this illness. The time has been interspersed with more doctor visits, medication trials and tests. After exploratory surgery, the urologist finally diagnosed a rare bladder disorder called interstitial cystitis. He detected scar tissue and hemorrhages in my bladder. This explains the almost constant searing pain. He says there is no cure for the condition. I read that some people with this disorder eventually become so desperate they resort to having their bladders removed. None of the doctors seem to think there is a connection between my bladder pain and the other symptoms. I do. They started at the same time, and a worsening of one often correlates with a worsening of the others.

A tube shoved down my throat into my stomach reveals that my esophagus is sore and inflamed. I'm told I have esophaghitis. Also, my rib cage is swollen and tender to the touch. Dr. Carson says it's an inflammation of the rib joints. On another visit, he noted that I had a slight fever and pleurisy. He is able to identify organic changes, but doesn't focus on or investigate causes. I looked up pleurisy in our medical guide at home. "Characterized by knife-like pains in the chest." They are the same kind of sharp, jabbing pains I've had moving around my chest since the onset of the illness. I believe that it must be what has been causing this discomfort all along. Looking up the causes of pleurisy, I find several—fungus infestation, pneumonia, cancer, toxoplasmosis. I read that toxoplasmosis is a disease transmitted by cats. It can be passed on to cattle and humans and occasionally results in chronic illness. We drink goats milk and I wonder if it is possible for goats to pass the organism to humans. I have our goats tested. They are positive, but my own blood tests come out negative.

I don't want to become a chronic complainer, but I'm afraid that Kim takes the brunt of whatever complaining I do. Nevertheless, he usually remains patient and consoling. At night when we get in bed we discuss my condition. "Whatever I've got, Kim, it seems to keep moving around my body. I've had inflammation of the bladder, inflammation of the esophagus, inflammation of the rib joints, inflammation of the lining of the lungs. Maybe I have inflammation of the brain, too. Somehow these symptoms must be connected. I never had any of them before 1981."

Kim has an external fungus that keeps moving around his body. He blames himself for my illness, convinced that he's passed the fungus on to me internally. He asks several doctors about it, but they say it's not very likely and would be pretty hard to prove. He is still sure that he's right.

LYME DISEASE: *My Search for a Diagnosis*

Mom is one hundred percent convinced that I have multiple sclerosis. From all the literature she's read, she says it fits.

I'm not sure of anything, except that I'm sick and I grasp at whatever comes along that might turn up a clue.

I am to keep grasping at straws for several years yet before I finally happen to catch one that produces some answers.

12

Through March 1984 - Calm before the storm

Kim and Jerimiah are getting ready to make their yearly trek to go deer hunting. I can never quite understand why they want to go way up by the Canadian border when we have deer practically in our back yard. Hunting on Mike's property they would probably have a better chance of getting a deer than they do up north. In fact the park behind us has opened to hunters for a few days because the deer population has increased to the nuisance level.

Jerimiah is so excited about going this year that he's been packing for a week. He and Kim have developed a close relationship. They are more than father and son; they have become buddies. I used to dread the hunting excursions, knowing they would be in the woods with so many other hunters and guns. And I was a big chicken when it came to staying home alone. But my worrying has never stopped them from going, so I've learned to put it out of my mind.

LYME DISEASE: *My Search for a Diagnosis*

It's even a relief when they're out the door and I'm no longer tripping over hunting gear, coolers, and sleeping bags.

This fall proves to be better than the past two. Van has moved out and, as much as we enjoyed him, it's nice to be back to our own family. The other children and I plan some visiting and manage to get an early start on Christmas shopping. My health seems considerably improved. In '81 I was too sick even to stay alone and Mary had come to stay with me. Last year I managed without her, but was in so much pain I was convinced that I didn't have long for this earth. Now I'm feeling the best I have in a long time. My gait still isn't normal, but it's not as obvious and my other symptoms are relatively mild. I've continued to take vitamins and my appetite is good. I'm working part time at a children's clothing shop. I've worked out a deal with the owner. I design and make clothing which I sell in her shop in exchange for tending the store and giving her a commission. I look forward to the days I work there. It's good to be out of the house and around people now that Jonathan is in school all day. Bobbi's dry humor appeals to me and we have fun working together.

* * *

Early in February, Kim comes home excited about some passes he can get from his brother Chuck, who works for an airline. We can both fly round trip to California for sixty dollars. I'm skeptical because we flew to the West Coast once before using this kind of pass and getting home became an enormous ordeal. "Come on, I really need to get away," Kim pleads. "We can have Mom and Bob stay with the kids, and Chuck says things should go smoother this time. We'll just go for a few days."

Calm before the storm

I hate asking people to look after the children when they've already put themselves out so much in the past years. I guess I feel more secure sticking close to home. Even though I have been feeling better, my bladder has been worse again lately.

Kim's persistence wins out and we are off on a 747 for Los Angeles. We are greeted by sun and balmy 70 degree weather. I have to admit it's a pleasant change from the sub-zero temperatures we left behind. From LA we drive down the coast to San Diego. We've been to this clean, friendly oceanside city once before with the children. The weather is almost perfect year-round.

As long as we've made the trip, I'm determined to spend some time at the beach and come back to Minnesota with a little color. Getting a tan isn't Kim's top priority, so it takes a little persuasion on my part to talk him into digging our swimsuits out of our suitcases the first morning and heading for a nearby beach before making other plans.

We find a niche among a cluster of boulders and spread our towels out to sit on. I read magazines while Kim strolls up and down the beach collecting shells to bring home to the children. When I'm tired of reading I watch the seagulls soaring high above, flapping their wings gracefully and swooping down when they spot a tourist strewing popcorn on the sand. I study the other vacationers sharing the beach with us. It's not hot enough to entice mobs of people out to sunbathe. There are only a few like us who have probably come from cooler climates and notice the contrast in temperature more.

By mid-day we're both getting bored and hungry and decide to head back to the hotel to change clothes. On the way we pick up fruit and crackers to snack on. I'm so hungry I devour a good share almost immediately.

At the hotel Kim goes up to our room while I linger outside to see where the pool is located. I am hoping to find a lounge chair and sneak in just a few more minutes of sun. As I walk across the pavement I can feel the warmth through the soles of my sandals. Rounding the corner of the building I catch a glimpse of sparkling turquoise blue. Suddenly my vision seems distorted and a sense of being out of touch with the surroundings overtakes me. I blink, trying to get things in focus and shake off the odd sensation. My heart begins racing—so fast it feels like it will fly out of my chest.

I have to find my way back to our room. I fumble my way back to the door, past the lobby. Room 312. I hope I remember the number right. I'm not sure that I'm going in the right direction. As I get on the elevator, a heavyset man is getting on with me. I feel like I'm getting weaker by the minute. Oh God, please don't let me lose it here. The elevator lurches to a stop and I stagger off, hoping I'm on the right floor. There's room 312. I can hear the TV. I knock feebly and Kim opens the door.

He looks alarmed. "What's wrong?"

"I don't know. Everything just got strange," I say, falling onto the bed, relieved to be free of the monumental effort it was taking to support my body.

Kim feels my head and checks my pulse. "Your hands are cold and clammy. Your heart feels like it's going 90 miles an hour!"

"I know. My chest hurts. It feels like there's a weight on it."

"I think we'd better call a doctor.

"Who would we call?" I ask weakly. "Just give me a little time to rest and see if it clears up." I feel so tired I don't want to move. So sleepy. The sound of Kim's voice and the TV set fade. I'm drifting into a peaceful place. Kim stays by my side shaking me and bringing me back out of the fog every few minutes. I mumble that I'm fine and drift off to sleep again.

Gradually things are becoming clearer and more focused. I sit up. "What time is it?"

Kim looks at his watch. "It's after seven. You've been like this for two hours. You really gave me a scare. Do you think you'll be okay to go out and get a bite to eat?"

"Yes, I think I'm fine now." I hope I am. I really don't want to mess up this vacation. Kim was looking forward to it so much. We eat sandwiches at a cafe, then drive around until we locate a shopping center.

"Mind if I stop at the department store and check out the men's shirts?" Kim asks.

"Sure, I need to look for a pair of shoes, too." I tag along with Kim, not quite trusting myself to venture off on my own. My bad leg is being more uncooperative than usual and it feels kind of twitchy. As Kim is talking to a sales clerk, the muscles in my leg are pulling so tightly that I can't control it and I'm forced to sit down on the floor to keep from falling. A lady with shopping bags walks by giving me a quizzical look and keeps walking. I know this looks strange but I can't help it.

Kim turns from the counter, spots me, and walks over. "Let's get out of here," he says gruffly. He pulls me up off the floor and half-carries me back out to the car. "I can see this is going to be a helluva vacation!"

After a night's sleep things seem to settle. We even spend half a day walking around the San Diego Zoo. As long as we stop to rest frequently I do fine. It still baffles me that this illness is so unpredictable, that my symptoms can come and go so suddenly.

The rest of the trip is spent browsing through the quaint gift and antique shops, picking up a few souvenirs for the children. We drive back to LA in time to spend an afternoon with Kim's Aunt Doris. She takes us out for seafood and insists on buying more mementos.

I'm grateful that the four-day excursion hasn't turned out all bad. I'm anxious to get home now. We called Minnesota to check on everything. Jerimiah had come home from school with the flu the day we left. I'm eager to see for myself that all is really okay.

When Kim calls the airport to check on the flight schedule it doesn't look promising. Things are really booked up. Normally there are plenty of openings in the middle of the week. We just happened to hit a bad time. They tell us we can come down and wait just in case there are cancellations.

We return our rental car. But things just aren't working out. The flight takes off without us and the next two days are booked solid. That will bring us to the weekend, and weekends are invariably busy. Our passes are classified lower than the usual standby tickets, which leaves the odds of getting on almost nil.

Kim needs to get back to work. Besides, staying in LA for four more days will be more expensive than paying full-fare to fly home on another airline. We concede and charge tickets on our credit card. Although we're disappointed, we agree it's the best option.

We have a six hour wait before our plane will leave. We haven't eaten and the airport food is ridiculously expensive. I suggest we flag down a shuttle bus and see if they'll be willing to drive us to a hotel just for a light meal.

We stand on the sidewalk until I spot a shuttle weaving in and out among the traffic. "Let's try that one," I say, noting that the name sounds inexpensive and casual. Kim waves his arm in the air to flag it down and the driver agrees to transport us for a meal and bring us back to the airport afterward. We begin to realize we've misjudged the casual sounding name as we climb into the van and notice the surroundings. The seats are upholstered in crimson velvet. The same plush fabric drapes the windows. The driver offers us a glass of champagne. After a short ride, he pulls up in front of our destination and ushers us through the classiest lobby I've ever seen, replete with massive crystal chandeliers, to an elegant formal dining room.

It's too late to turn back now. We stand sheepishly in our blue jeans and tennis shoes with duffle bags slung over our shoulders, staring at people in tuxedos and formal gowns who are all politely ignoring us.

A sophisticated waiter escorts us to a velvet-draped booth and pulls the curtains nearly shut. He seems as embarrassed as we are. He peers between the curtains and asks if we'd like to order drinks. When he leaves, Kim and I look at each other exploding into laughter. "What the heck, we might as well go all out," he exclaims. "Why, they don't even have prices on the menu! I'll just charge it!"

The incident provides an entertaining story to relate to the family when we get home. However, we both decide this is the last good deal we'll take advantage of for a long time! Our humorous mood, the trip, in fact the past several months turn out to be the eye of calm in the center of a storm. The violent raging hurricane, the worst period of our six-year struggle with my unknown illness, it yet to come.

Wait on the Lord:
be of good courage, and
he shall strengthen thine heart
Psalms 27:14

13

March 1984 - My alien body

In the first week home after our Califirnia trip I had two more spells similar to the one I had outside the hotel in San Diego—the same visual distortion, racing heart, extreme weakness, followed by sleepiness. One happened in church and the whole service was disrupted as people scurried to help me. The other occurred at Bobbi's shop. She was there at the time and it scared her to death. She immediately phoned her own doctor. He came right to the shop and picked me up off the floor as though I were a limp rag doll, carried me to his car and drove me to his nearby clinic. I thought it was rather gallant of him. He kept me under observation until my strength began to come back, but he too was baffled as to the cause of the spell. He urged me to contact my own doctor and to consider seeing a heart specialist. I put it off. The past two-and-a-half years' experience with doctors hasn't given me any confidence that

LYME DISEASE: My Search for a Diagnosis

they'll be able to find the source of the problem, let alone to correct it. Bobbi has become skittish about having me watch the store alone and Kim is nervous, too. "You're going to have to stay home until we find out what's going on. I can't be worrying about you every time you leave the house," he scolds.

Reluctantly I call Dr. Carson back. He suggests that my spells might be seizure-related and asks me to set up an appointment with Dr. Steele.

It's a few days before my appointment and Kim and I are sitting in the TV room. I'm working on some hand sewing. It feels like another spell is coming on. My heart is racing and when I look up the TV screen is out of focus. Oh Lord, please—if I ignore this maybe it'll go away. But the muscles in the calf of my right leg are pulling my foot inward and my leg is lifting itself off the floor independently of any conscious instruction from my brain. It's as though the leg has decided to become a separate unit and chooses to have a will of its own.

"Kim, look at this. My leg is doing this by itself. It's weird. I can't put it down."

Kim peers quizzically at my leg, which is sticking straight out from the chair, my right foot pulled tightly inward.

"My head feels funny, like it's too heavy for my shoulders."

"Maybe you'd better lie down," Kim says, as he lifts me out of the chair and stretches me out on the carpet. The muscles in the right side of my trunk are pulling now too, wrenching my body violently to the right side in quick motions and my right leg is jerking crazily.

Kim isn't panicking; he just looks flustered. "You stay here. I'm going to call Dr. Carson."

My alien body

I can hear parts of the conversation. I gather that Dr. Carson is at the hospital waiting to deliver a baby. They discuss the situation for a long time before Kim comes back and relates that Dr. Carson doesn't think it's necessary to bring me to the hospital. "He says that maybe this is the hard neurological symptom they've been waiting for in order to diagnose your illness, but it should be okay to wait till you see Dr. Steele."

"That's not for three days. Isn't there anything we can do now? I'm not real excited about staying like this."

"He suggested that sometimes a change of position helps. Why don't we try to get you up off the floor and see if a warm bath will help relax you."

With Kim's help I can walk—bizarrely, haltingly, unsure how to deal with this body that seems to have become a creature apart from me.

He draws some warm bath water and helps me undress and get in. I watch the water slosh and swirl around my body with the now almost rhythmic convulsive movement. Kim sits on the edge of the tub, rubbing his face with his hands. Emotionally, I feel nothing. I think we're both numb, so used to strange things happening that we barely react anymore.

The bath doesn't help still my muscles. Kim tucks me into bed. I'm feeling so tired again that I have no trouble drifting off to sleep. Fragments of thoughts float to my consciousness. A diagnosis—Dr. Carson sounded hopeful—That'd be great after two and a half years—Maybe this is a dream—When I wake up it'll be gone—and I can forget about this nonsense.

But, the next morning as soon as I'm fully awake the movement resumes. I get up and make my way to the kit-

LYME DISEASE: My Search for a Diagnosis

chen feeling like I'm trying to do an uncoordinated jig. Jenny and Jonathan, who have already come downstairs, are wide-eyed at first, a bit in shock.

"Mom! What's the matter with you?" Jenny questions.

"I don't know yet. I have a doctor's appointment in a few days. Maybe I'll find something out. Dr. Carson seems to think this might mean a diagnosis."

"Oh Mom, I hope so!" Jenny exclaims.

They continue to stare, looking like they aren't sure whether to laugh or cry. When they see my calmness, they decide it must not be too serious. Jenny puts her hand over her mouth, trying to stifle a giggle. "I'm sorry Mom, but you look really funny. You look like a chicken when you walk."

"She looks like she's trying to dance," Jonathan pipes in.

We all break out in giggles then as I make my way around the kitchen and begin to fix pancakes. At least I have complete control in my arms so I'll be able to stay busy.

Jerimiah and Jason seem to react coolly to the new situation. Years later Jerimiah tells me that he didn't know what to think and found that he had to leave the room. Jennifer will eventually spill out much pent up emotion and fear.

14

The unspoken message on Dr. Steele's face as he enters the exam room and sees my contortions can't be any clearer. He might as well say it out loud. He thinks I'm making this up. He actually thinks I'm making this up! I wonder if he can read my mind, my dismay, as clearly as I can read his skepticism.

He shakes his head. "I've just never seen anything like this before—Of course, I've seen a lot of pretty unusual things—I suppose we'd better repeat some of the tests. There's a chance that a seizure disorder could cause something like this although I doubt it. I don't expect anything to show up on the tests—I still think this is a psychosomatic problem."

I've gotten my hopes up for nothing. There isn't going to be a diagnosis. Why did I let myself think there ever could be? I need to keep my composure. "I'd have to be more than slightly neurotic to come up with symptoms like these."

Dr. Steele nods. "You're right."

"But if I am such a basket case you'd think my family and friends would have realized it, even if I can't see it. But they don't believe that either."

He shrugs. "I don't know."

"All right, if this is all the result of some monumental psychological problem, what am I supposed to do about it?" I ask in exasperation.

"It may take years of psychotherapy and you have to be willing to be helped before anyone can help you," he replies.

I'm devastated by his answer. After two and a half years of praying that I'd be taken seriously, not seen as a victim of my own hysteria, I'm back where I started. I tell myself to stay calm. My anger is not going to help.

I am scheduled for tests again and before I leave Dr. Steele writes out a prescription that he says will help control the jerking.

I don't want Kim to see how discouraged I am. How long will he keep believing in me? I don't think I can face going back to Dr. Steele. I know that I need to do something, but I don't see how I can justify spending hundreds, maybe thousands, of dollars we don't have on psychoanalysis, trying to find a problem that I can't believe exists.

On the way home Kim stops at the drugstore for my prescription. I smooth out the slip which I've wadded up in my fist and hand it to him. "Ask the pharmacist for a pamphlet on the drug, too, would you?"

I've learned from experience that the pamphlets issued by the drug companies are usually more informative than the books on prescription drugs. I'm surprised that the drug Dr. Steele prescribed is an anti-seizure medication. If he's so sure that my problem isn't real, how could he have been so confident this medication will work? Maybe it's just a placebo. However, I take it and within a few days the movement is almost totally subdued. My other symptoms aren't helped though. The pain is bad, I'm running a slight fever and I'm waking up again at night drenched in sweat.

My friend Lois has a brother who is a neurologist. She's mentioned several times that he's an excellent diagnostician. I've balked at going to him in the past because the thought of a friend's brother telling me I was neurotic was too threatening.

I've decided to make an appointment with him and if he is as convinced as Dr. Steele that my problems are in my psyche, I'll concede. I'll go for counseling and somehow find a way to pay for it. I don't know what else to do.

Kim says whatever I decide to do is fine. I can see that he's having a rough time now. He just wants to tune out. I try not to take his apparent coolness personally. It seems that every time we start getting caught up financially, the medical bills start piling up again. I feel like I'm on an emotional roller coaster that never stops.

* * *

After many persistent phone calls I'm finally able to make an appointment with Lois's brother, Dr. Schut. He only sees patients one-half day a week because he spends most of his time on research. His nurse kept telling me he wasn't taking any new patients, but I've finally gotten in. He wants me to get copies of Aunt Anne's records. I'm impressed that he's considering my genetic history. I've mentioned Aunt Anne to a few other doctors, but no one else has shown much interest. At least Dr. Schut is going to be thorough. Ever since the beginning Aunt Anne has been in the back of my mind. Maybe at least I will find out if there is any connection between our illnesses.

Aunt Anne and Uncle Ed have both passed away, but through my great uncles in Florida I am able to obtain information and locate the hospital where Aunt Anne was treated. It is easy to get copies of her medical records by sending a small fee along with a signed release from the next of kin.

When the records arrive in a thick brown envelope, I tear them open, more than a little curious as to what I might find. As I skim them, I can't help picking out some similarities between her illness and mine. The records cover a span of time from her early thirties till her death at fifty-eight. I flip through the pages of history, test results, impressions, and diagnoses, then reread them slowly. I discover, to my surprise, that there actually was a name given her disease—syringomyelia. I'd been told her disease had never been diagnosed. The age of onset was close to mine. Hers was heralded by difficulty walking. At some .point she also had numbness in her face and bladder problems. And as near as I can translate from the medical jargon, there had even been some jerking muscle spasms.

My stomach is churning. I feel like I'm going to vomit. For the first time in almost three years of searching for an answer, a feeling of panic grips me. From the description, I envision Aunt Anne lying utterly helpless, her body contorted in painful spasms. Not only was she almost totally paralyzed, her head was fixed permanently to one side, and one leg became twisted in an awkward angle.

Angrily, I fling the papers down on my bed. I've known all

these years that she suffered, but the reality of the depth of her pain portrayed in her records is overwhelming. I bury my head in a pillow and sob uncontrollably for a long time. It just isn't fair that she had to suffer the way she did for so many years. I cry for Aunt Anne, for everyone who has to endure disease and pain, and for myself.

When I finally run out of tears I feel completely drained, like I have been turned inside out and stripped of any feeling. I pick up the records and stuff them back into the envelope, deliberately forcing the images they created out of my mind. I refuse to have anything as morbid and pathetic as Aunt Anne had. I won't give in to this illness. At least I can still get up and function more often than not, and I have my family. Aunt Anne's only pregnancy had ended in a miscarriage.

I bring Aunt Anne's records with me to my appointment with Dr. Schut. By now I have managed to disassociate myself from them. Lois told me I would like her brother and I do immediately. He has a disarming personality and a broad, friendly grin. After looking over Aunt Anne's medical records he assures me that syringomyelia is not what I have.

Concerning my mental status he says, "I don't think you're any more neurotic than the rest of us, probably less so." He notes that I have swollen glands, and because of my night sweats he decides to refer me to an infectious disease specialist.

Another doctor! I had no idea there were so many different areas of specialty within the medical profession.

* * *

LYME DISEASE: My Search for a Diagnosis

Dr. Christian Schrock, the new specialist, brings up another possiblity. "Has anyone ever tested you for lupus?" he asks.

"I don't know if they have or not." Most of the doctors I've seen don't tell me anything they are checking for unless I pry it out of them.

Several more vials of blood are drawn.

At home, I pull out my trusty medical guide. Lupus. Systemic Lupus Erythematosus...generalized inflammatory disorder affecting connective tissues. Young adult females most frequently affected. No consistent pattern order...Pleurisy common...May be manifested in one or several organ systems....

My symptoms seem to fit. But the blood work comes back inconclusive. Dr. Schrock says it indicates the possibility of lupus, but there's not enough evidence to make a diagnosis. What else is new?

He and Dr. Schut agree that some sort of collagen vascular disease related to lupus is the most likely culprit. Collagen diseases fall into the category of rheumatic disorders. He prescribes anti-inflammatory medication. Is this the answer to my strange and varying array of symptoms? Even though I still have no concrete answers, it's comforting to have doctors who don't appear to be discounting my problems. They make my predicament a whole lot easier to deal with.

15

August 1984 - My own shop

I have always dreamed of having a sewing shop of my own but the illness has destroyed my confidence.There are times when I think I could handle it, if it weren't for these maddeningly unpredictable symptoms.

I'd really given up on the idea, but a phone call from an acquaintance in town has rekindled the dream. Maxine, another local seamstress, called today suggesting we consider opening a shop together. She even knows of a space for rent in Delano.

The call has come at a good time. After a rough July, my health seems to be on an upswing. I find myself agreeing to go look at the rental space located behind the beauty shop on Main Street. To say that the place needs a complete overhaul is a grand understatement. The affordable rent tempts us both into envisioning a cheery work area beyond the debris and filth. After talking it over with our husbands,

LYME DISEASE: My Search for a Diagnosis

Maxine and I decide to go for it. She knows I've had health problems, but is willing to risk the venture.

I can't help believing that God has opened up this opportunity for me. Things seem to fall into place. Maxine and I easily agree on the wallpaper, paint and carpeting. I watch her plunge energetically into the rejuvenation project. Her drive reminds me of my own before the illness.

Maxine is about my height, just a smidgen over five feet and of sturdy build. As I watch her work, I think to myself that at one time I would have been able to match her zeal. I'm thankful, however, to be able to contribute a reasonable amount of assistance in the scrubbing, dry wall taping, and painting. In fact, I am surprised at how much I am able to do. We recruit our spouses to help. Maxine's husband, Lowell, is a carpenter. With their combined skills, he and Kim put in a new ceiling, install dry wall, section off areas for dressing rooms and lay carpeting.

A few weeks later The Sew It All Shop is ready for finishing touches—a ruffled skirt to hide the ugly pipes under the bathroom sink, throw pillows for the blue loveseat I brought from home, curtains for the dressing room doors and we're ready for our grand opening.

We aren't quite prepared for the avalanche of business that immediately fills our shop. We haven't even had to advertise. Through the fall we both work full-time and hire occasional helpers. Our arrangement is ideal. We each specialize in different types of sewing, she in alterations and I in knitwear, so we aren't in competition.

Maxine has a more aggressive personality than I do, but we blend well together. We seem to complement each other both in sewing skills and personality traits.

Things go so well that health concerns are almost forgotten until late December when I have a spell again similar to those of a year earlier. After Christmas, orders come in more slowly, so Maxine and I tackle a couple of joint projects. But the spells start coming more frequently. The uncontrollable jerking movement is back. This time it's accompanied by twisting head motions. At first it's intermittent and I try to continue working in spite of it.

When I see Dr. Schrock he is able to observe the peculiarity that I have only been able to describe to him in the past. "Maybe we should admit you to the hospital and see if we can get to the bottom of this," he suggests.

Traveling down the long tunnel leading from the clinic to the hospital, I attract side glances from passersby with my odd contortions and strange gait. I don't want to let my mind race too far ahead and start getting my hopes up, but for some reason I have good feelings about this appointment. Maybe something positive will come of it.

A woman at the admitting desk hands me forms to fill out and when I finish I'm instructed to wait for a neurologist that Dr. Schrock has arranged for me to see. In a short time, I spot a man with silver-white hair and slightly hunched shoulders walking briskly towards me. As he approaches, he reaches out with a warm handshake. "You must be Linda Hanner. I'm Dr. John Witek."

As he ushers me into a nearby exam room, there is a gentleness in his manner that puts me more at ease than any doctor I've seen. He listens with interest as I recite the almost four-year-saga that I've repeated so many times by now I've almost memorized it.

"I realize this must be terribly frustrating for you," he comments when I finish. "This has been going on long enough that you deserve some answers. I sure hope we'll be able to come up with some for you."

It's the first time a doctor has verbally empathized with my predicament. I am encouraged by this man who seems so thoughtful and so determined to help.

By the time I'm settled in a room it's past dinner. A meal is arranged. The nurse has been instructed by Dr. Schrock to spoon feed me and they have padded the sides of my bed. Apparently Dr. Schrock is concerned about the possibility of symptoms progressing to a full-blown seizure. I feel a little silly, yet I appreciate the concern after so often being met with indifference by other doctors.

The nurses are shorthanded and extra busy tonight. The curtains on the window are drawn, but from the TV weather reports I learn that the snow that was falling lightly when I came in is turning into near blizzard conditions. The medication they prescribe is making me groggy.

* * *

The next morning, I just finish brushing my teeth and combing my hair when Dr. Witek arrives. As he appraises the situation for a minute, I'm struck that his kind, clear blue eyes perfectly match the sweater he is wearing. "One thing I'm sure of is that there is an organic explanation to your symptoms. If there isn't, you deserve an academy award," he announces.

He doesn't know how much his complete and immediate faith in that fact means to me. Now I am convinced that he was sent directly from heaven.

"Does your movement stop when you're sleeping?"

"Yes, as far as I know."

"That's pretty typical. Most movement disorders settle

down when you're relaxed or sleeping. And by the way, it's very common for them to be more exaggerated when you're out in public. Some of my patients with Parkinson's disease complain that their tremors aren't present at home, but immediately start up when they go out and there is more stimulation."

This information that Dr. Witek is taking time to volunteer is significant. My movement does act up more when I'm away from home. I know Kim is aware of it too and even though he doesn't say it, I'm afraid that he thinks I'm manipulating to get attention.

I am deeply impressed with this doctor. And I pray that he and Dr. Schrock together will be able to solve my mysterious illness. However, between now and the answer to that prayer there will stretch a long period of almost complete despair.

Aside from trying to uncover the cause of my symptoms, Dr. Witek and Dr. Schrock's main concern is to get my movement, which they now are defining as chorea, under control.

One afternoon, when I get out of bed and stand up the chorea goes completely wild. My back arches, the muscles in my side pull violently, my legs are uncontrollable. Two nurses arrive and it requires a good deal of effort with them working together to guide me back to bed. The smaller blond one teases, "This isn't so bad. I had a 200 pound guy fall on me one time. He pinned me right against the wall. Thank goodness you're as small as you are."

I grip the rails of the bed trying to control the writhing. "I feel so agitated. Dr. Witek prescribed a different drug today. Do you think it could be from the medication?" I ask.

The dark-haired nurse responds to my question, "One of

the possible side effects of the drug is agitation, although most people respond the opposite way. I'll call Dr. Witek and see what he wants us to do." She returns bringing me a tranquilizer to counteract the effects of the first drug. It makes me doze the rest of the evening and when my family comes I can barely stay awake long enough to follow the conversation. Yet, underneath, I still feel a driving restlessness.

By the fourth day in the hospital I'm fighting feelings of discouragement that are creeping in to replace my earlier optimism. All the testing has again failed to reveal any definite answers. I hate the way these drugs are making me feel. It's more difficult to tolerate their effects than the chorea. I feel like climbing the walls.

When I see Dr. Witek I ask him to take me off the medication. He agrees and he and Dr. Schrock release me from the hospital that day. They still seem to think I must have some sort of collagen vascular disorder, but no specific one is identified, nor do I have a treatment plan.

I am dressed and waiting for Mom and Dad to come and pick me up when a lab technician rushes into my room, carrying a clattering tray of vials. "We need to take some more blood before you leave."

"What for?" I ask wearily. It seems that enough blood has been drained from my system by now to provide for a lifetime of tests.

"Dr. Schrock wants to check for something called Lyme disease."

I have no idea what this is. I look under "Lime" and find nothing on it in the medical books at home or the library. It must be a real long shot, whatever it is. Anyway, next time I

My own shop

see Dr. Schrock he tells me the tests have all come back negative, so I promptly forget about it.

He who believes in me, as the scripture has said,
'Out of his heart shall flow rivers of living water'
John 7:38 RSV

16

February 1985 - New treatments

I return to work at the shop in spite of the fact that the chorea isn't under control. Often I don't have the stamina to make it through the day, so I lay down on the dressing room floor to rest.

People react to me in different ways when the jerking is most noticeable. Some simply avoid looking at me and pretend I'm invisible. Most respond well. I never mind people asking questions, expressing their own dismay at seeing me this way. Those who voice their feelings usually are accepting and go on to treat me as always. Those who express compassion and concern, but don't dwell on the problem, are the most helpful to me.

During times when my gait becomes more extreme in its awkwardness, Maxine nicknames me "Lurch." Her ability to make light of the situation in spite of her genuine concern makes it easy to continue working with her at the shop.

LYME DISEASE: *My Search for a Diagnosis*

Kim has a harder time dealing with the movement than he has any of my other symptoms. I sense that it's difficult for the children too, especially in public. Jonathan has said more than once, "I wish you weren't like this, Mom."

Anytime there is a lot of visual or audio stimulation around me the movement becomes more exaggerated. When I attend church, school plays, and band concerts the movement may be pretty subdued on arrival, but by the time we are ready to leave the muscles in my body are pulling and jerking against each other so hard that it's difficult to walk back to the car. At first Kim wants to hustle me out as soon as he can see the tension in my face as I try to concentrate with little avail on keeping my body still. Only once does someone make the remark, "Why doesn't Linda just stay home if she doesn't feel good?" If I stay home every time I don't feel well, I will become a hermit. I need to be out and around people. Most of my friends do encourage me to get out and their encouragement eventually helps Kim to become more comfortable with the situation, too.

Dr. Schrock seems surprised that I can work. I tell him that I do fine, but avoid the use of my electric cutter. He and Dr. Witek discuss medications again and finally decide to try me on Thorazine, a major tranquilizer that sometimes is used in treating movement disorders. In order for it to become effective, I need to take such a high dose that I become zombie-like and can barely function.

I call Dr. Witek when I note my speech is becoming halting at times. He says it makes sense because the same part of my brain that controls movement also controls speech. Dr. Witek and I also explore the possibility of poisoning from garden dust. While I was still in the hospital he had asked if I ever used rose dust. I don't have roses, but recall that the summer I became ill I went through several canisters of garden dust to prevent the bugs from demolishing my vegetables. Dr. Witek and I both contact the manufacturer and are informed that the product I used is capable of causing neurological symptoms if absorbed through the skin or ingested. However, the company chemist also assures us that the body eventually will rid itself of the poison and symptoms would have cleared up within a few months. Another dead end.

* * *

On February 12 I am scheduled to speak at our local Christian Business and Professional Women's Club luncheon. I worked on my testimony for a long time and am excited that I have been approved as a speaker. In spite of the fact that my symptoms are so active, I don't consider cancelling the engagement. I have strong feelings that I am meant to do this.

Many people are praying for me the day the luncheon rolls around and the prayers must be getting through. In the morning my chorea is barely detectable. I need to sit during my half-hour talk because my balance is off, otherwise I make it through beautifully. My speech poses no problems, and as unusual as it is for my movement to be still in public, it remains under control throughout. I'm pleased. Most of my life I've been an introvert and getting up in front of a group would have been worse than jumping off a bridge, but now I enjoy sharing and the audience responds enthusiastically to my talk. Mainly, I'm happy about the opportunity to share my faith in a loving, caring God, in spite of life's problems. I am invited to speak at another area luncheon in March.

LYME DISEASE: My Search for a Diagnosis

A few days after the speaking engagement, Dr. Schrock suggests trying me on Prednisone, which is a steroid. At this point I'm game. The movement has been active most of the time for over a month and it hasn't been easy on us. None of the other medication tried has been effective and from what I've heard, Prednisone has produced dramatic results in a wide variety of ailments. Dr. Schrock explains that I won't be able to stay on it for long and will have to gradually taper to a lower dose.

The first week of the treatment I'm almost high. I'm not sure how much is from the drug itself and how much is because I'm so thrilled to be feeling this good. All my symptoms have disappeared. I have energy. I'd forgotten what it's like to feel this well. Other people have warned me that they've become depressed going off this type of drug, but I'm not overly concerned. I've been depressed before, and knowing it's a side effect from the drug should help. Nothing on earth could prepare me for what actually happens.

17

March 1985 - Plunging into the pit

The first time I notice anything awry, I am working at the shop. As lunchtime nears, an intense, bizarre feeling of hopelessness and despair descends out of nowhere. It hovers for about an hour, then disappears as mysteriously as it came.

The next day there are more episodes like it. One moment I feel perfectly normal, the next I'm hurled into a strange dark pit where everything is distorted and threatening. When I call Dr. Schrock to tell him how frightened I am he instructs me to go back to my original dose of the Prednisone. I assume he thinks it will balance my system again. Each day the episodes become more frequent and last longer, gradually becoming an almost constant haunting companion.

I try to describe to Kim what is happening and he can't absorb it, yet he can see by the terror-stricken look in my eyes that something is drastically wrong. I stop sleeping at night, too agitated to stay in bed. As soon as I hear Kim's slow, raspy breathing indicating he's asleep, I get up and roam from one room to the next. The chorea has resumed, but it's insignificant compared to my mental agony.

Sometimes I pause in front of the window and gaze out into the night at the shadowed tree branches. Or I stand looking at my reflection in the bathroom mirror. The face that stares back has an anguished, inhuman quality. I feel disconnected from it. I pace some more, running my hand along the walls, touching the furniture, frantically trying to feel in contact with the world I was a part of. Terror is gripping and consuming me. I cry to God aloud in a hollow voice, "Please help me find a way out of this nightmare!" My cries seem to fall on emptiness. I wander to the bathroom again and open the medicine chest, pulling out a package of razor blades. I stare at them and slowly place them back on the top shelf. My actions and thoughts seem to be coming from a foreboding source not a part of my being.

Kim calls Dr. Schrock once more to report my extreme distress and he finally decides I should discontinue the drug gradually. I remain in the nightmare. Oh God, please let there be an end to this. Dr. Schrock said it will take three days before the medication is out of my system. If I can just hang on until then.

The first day, a Friday evening, Kim needs to make a cabinet delivery near Mom and Dad's house. "Linda, I don't think you should stay here alone. Come with me and I'll drop you off at your mom's."

Being confined in the car is pure torture. Yet existing in open spaces from moment to moment feels equally punishing.

Plunging into the pit

When I see Mom I clutch her tightly, like a frightened child. We sit in the living room. There is a seldom-used softness in her voice as she talks, the way she sounded whenever I was sick as a young girl. I try to concentrate on her voice in hopes it will draw me back into the world which for me is fragmenting.

Kim returns, and when Mom asks him to leave me with her for the night he seems relieved. After he goes, she fixes a makeshift bed on the living room floor with sheets and blankets and stays by me through the night, talking and holding me. At times my body jerks uncontrollably. Her labor of love pales compared to the horrors going on inside myself.

A strangely muffled roaring occupies my head accompanied by visions of blood and knives. I try desperately to drown the horror by filling my conscious mind with Bible verses. Mom is quoting, "This too shall pass." But I am consumed in terror, crushed—forsaken by God.

The night passes. On Saturday Mom leaves my side only long enough to get meals for Dad. She is afraid to leave me alone. I'm becoming preoccupied with finding a way of escape from this madness. In the early morning hours of Sunday I manage to lie still long enough for Mom to think I am sleeping. She gets up and I hear her footsteps fade in the direction of her bedroom. She needs some rest. I'm compelled by an indefinable force to get up from my pallet and walk through the moonlit dining room into the kitchen. The blue lilies that Mom painted on the cupboard doors when I was a child are still there, but the white painted background has yellowed over the years. I pull open a drawer and take out a long knife. The roaring creates an all-consuming pressure in my head.

LYME DISEASE: *My Search for a Diagnosis*

An evil stranger to myself, I drag the glistening blade across my wrist applying just enough pressure to scratch the surface of the skin. Again and again I repeat the action, first over the left wrist, then the right. Only scratches appear, with a hint of red beginning to ooze from them.

I hear footsteps and Mom's voice calling my name. She is standing here watching me return the knife to the drawer.

"You couldn't do it, could you?" she is saying. "It'll be okay, Linda. It'll be okay."

But soon it will be the third day and this living horror isn't lifting.

Later on, I hear Mom and Dad's muffled conversation. "We should take her to the hospital," Dad says.

Mom replies, "I'm scared they'll just put her on more medication. If she can just get this out of her system, I'm sure she'll be better."

On Sunday I sit, stare, jerk, and pace. The inner tumult is no less intense. I haven't slept in four nights. I have to pull out of this today or I know my spirit will be doomed to stay forever in this diabolic place. But I can't. Just do something normal. I can't. I'm insane. Somehow I need to feign sanity—convince Mom and Dad I'm better. I can't stay here anymore, can't keep putting them through this hell with me.

Mom is putting a bowl of sliced peaches in front of me. Somehow I manage to force them down. In the afternoon they agree to bring me home.

As forms of trees and houses whiz by the car window, I fight the urge to open the car door and fling myself to the pavement. I feel so unspeakably sick—not physically ill, but destroyed in my mind, a wretched mind-sickness.

Kim and the children are watching TV when we get to our house. It's almost five o'clock. I can't let them see my in-

Plunging into the pit

sanity. I keep my sleeves pulled low over my wrists to hide the scratches.

I tell myself to start supper, take the electric fry pan down from the cupboard and reach for some meat from the freezer. Mom and Dad are saying good-bye, telling us to be sure and call if we need them. I'm holding a package of steak in my hand, but I can't go any further. I'm immobilized. My body doesn't respond to the directions I give it. This craziness is controlling me.

Kim reaches over and takes the meat out of my hands. "Linda, just go to bed. You need to sleep. I'll take care of this."

He takes my arm and guides me to the bedroom, shutting the door behind me. I'm engulfed by the dark, but no physical darkness can begin to match the blackness penetrating the depths of my soul. It's the end of the third day and I am trapped helplessly in a hell within myself.

I hear shuffling steps pass by the door. There is silence in the direction of the kitchen. The TV is on in the family room. Quietly I slip out of the bedroom and shut the door carefully behind me. In the bathroom I find the razor blades resting on the top shelf. Once again I pull them down. Clutching the package, I steal through the back entryway and down the steps to our basement. I crouch by the crumbling concrete of the back wall. Every motion seems logical now. I pray incoherently as I stare at the drops of blood forming a puddle on the painted maroon floor. The pressure of the blade brings no pain. The sight of blood, which has always made me queasy, now brings a curious sense of relief.

*Terrors are turned upon me: they
pursue my soul as the wind: and my
welfare passeth away as a cloud*
Job 30:15

18

March 1985 Continued - Falling further

"You didn't really want to hurt yourself. You were just trying to ask for help, weren't you?" Dr. Schrock is saying as he examines my wrists.

It hadn't been a plea for help. Had I believed that anyone could help, I wouldn't have done it. They had all tried to help me. Nothing had worked. No one can help. I hadn't wanted to hurt myself or even just to die. I had wanted to wipe out my miserable existence—never to have existed at all. There is no way I can make anyone understand that.

What had made Kim decide to leave the television program and look for me the night before?

His eyes had been full of fire when he found me. Pulling me roughly up the stairs, he seethed, "We're not going to tell the kids. We just *can't* let them know." After binding my wrists with towels, he shoved my arms into my coat sleeves and yanked me to the car. He headed for the larger downtown hospital. First there was tortured silence as he drove, then abruptly it was broken by a stream of profanity. In the twenty years I'd known Kim, I'd never heard him use that kind of language.

"I'm through praying," he snarled. "From now on I'm not having anything to do with God." His words, uttered with terrible anger, felt like a thousand knives cutting through my soul. It was unbearable that not only had God apparently turned His back on me, but that because of my own wretched state Kim was giving up on his faith too.

When we arrived at the emergency room I spotted a woman in the lobby who had wandered in off the street—a disheveled, glassy-eyed form, probably a drug addict. Sunken eyes, straggled hair, rumpled dress, her body twitching oddly, not unlike my own. I couldn't take my eyes off her. I was revolted, yet in her pitiful state I saw what I perceived to be a reflection of myself.

A doctor in the emergency room had examined me, stating that my present situation was probably caused by a combination of the effects of the drug and the unnamed illness that had called for using it. When he learned that I'd been under the care of doctors who practiced at a suburban hospital he thought it best to send us there. He dressed and bandaged my wounds. Only superficial cuts, he had said. Having to drive across town didn't help to calm Kim's fury.

The last thing I remembered after arriving was an emergency room aide walking over to the cart I was on and asking me what had happened. I was unable to make my mouth form any words to respond to his question. Another attendant came with a needle, and everything went blank.

When I came to again it was morning. A high-pitched voice filled with despair greeted me from across the room.

Falling further

Its owner was a woeful creature—merely a girl, who was scratching her arms viciously as she spoke. "I'm allergic to the carpeting up here." Every visible part of her body was covered with an angry red rash. "They're going to move me downstairs today," she prattled.

* * *

When Dr. Schrock is gone I begin rummaging through my purse. The nurses at the desk had removed a mirror earlier, but overlooked a seam ripper. I shut myself in the bathroom and pull off the cloth wrapped around my wrists, but a nurse is tapping on the door, and I shove the seam ripper under the sink as she enters. She scolds me for removing the bandages and goes to fetch more cloth and tape to redo them.

I wander out of my room down the hospital corridor till I come to a door leading to a shower stall. I pull off my sweater and jeans, step into the cold cubicle and turn on the nozzle full force. I slam my body against the ceramic wall and claw at the tile with my fingers as the hot water streams over me. There is no distraction from the agony. No distraction at all. When I step out again there is no towel. I pull my clothes back on over my wet body. The new bandages on my wrists are soaked through.

In the corridor I spot a swarthy complexioned doctor walking toward me. "Please—help me," I implore. "Please."

"I'll be in to see you in awhile. Just stay in your room and wait," he says stonily as he continues to walk down the hall. When he returns, he throws some questions at me. His eyes seem cold and lifeless, his voice without expression. Then he goes to order medication—an antidepressant, two kinds of tranquilizers, and a hypnotic drug for sleeping. I'm fright-

LYME DISEASE: My Search for a Diagnosis

ened. It was a drug that triggered this nightmare in the first place. Now I have become a victim and prisoner of drugs.

All the drugs combined barely subdue the torment, which is intensified by the realization of what I have done to myself—tried to do. It was as good as doing it. Fate. It is just fate that I am still here walking around. Nothing can ever, ever be the same again now. Why has God turned a deaf ear to my cries? I try to think of the Bible verses I had memorized in our Bible study. I was told they would help me during difficult times.

God is faithful, who will not suffer you to be tempted above what ye are able; but will...also make a way to escape, that ye may be able to bear it (I Corinthians 10:13). But I am not able to bear it. There had been no way of escape. The verse has proved meaningless. It is done now, over, no way to go back and fix it. I can never face my Christian friends again.

Was it barely two months ago that I was so confident in my faith that I spoke at a Christian Women's Luncheon, sharing my belief in a loving, caring God, a God who answers prayers? If I had lifted anyone up with that talk it is now more than destroyed. How many others will I drag into this abyss with me? Oh God, why did you let me get to the point that I was so certain of your love that I wanted to share it? It would have been better to have kept silent.

A nurse is poking her head in the door of my room. "Come on. It's time for the exercise group to start."

I don't respond, don't move. She comes over and takes my arm firmly, "Come on now, you have to go down there." She escorts me to a room at the other end of the hall. Chairs have been pushed to the outer walls. A tape cassette is blaring its lively music. A group of patients, some still in ill-fitting cot-

- 110 -

Falling further

ton pajamas and pin-striped hospital robes, are gathered in
the center of the room.

"One, two, three, four—That's it, now take a deep
breath," a sweatsuit-clad nurse is saying. I walk to the corner in the back and watch. A young man in front of me is
swinging to the music, singing out loud. I make a few feeble
attempts at imitating the moving bodies. My arms and legs
are lead weight, a strangling sensation fills my chest and
throat. I just want to run away, disappear. But I can't
escape. The fear, the strangling sensation will be with me no
matter how far I run.

Group therapy occupies the rest of the morning. I sit
rigidly in my chair, forming part of the circle of bodies.
Somebody is talking—a woman's voice drones on endlessly.

When I come back to my room, my roommate is gone.
They've taken her to a different floor. A new patient is being
brought in, a tiny-boned young woman with fragile features,
meticulously groomed.

"That psychiatrist. I didn't like him. He was only here
five minutes," she whimpers. "I came here because I was
afraid I was going to kill myself. It's this hairdo. I came
home after having it permed and when I looked in the mirror
I just freaked out. Do you think it's awful?"

"No, I think it looks nice."

Nothing seems to be making any sense.

Later in the day, it is time for occupational therapy. I
don't want to go but again the nurse is here, prodding and
insisting.

"Oh God, I feel like I'm going to suffocate," I think as I
enter a room filled with activity. Patients are painting, glu-
ing, pounding. A therapist shows me drawers full of beads,
rope, leather, and wooden scraps.

LYME DISEASE: My Search for a Diagnosis

"What do you want to work on today?"
I just want to leave—it is all meaningless. It is all crazy
and I am crazy. The walls feel like they're closing in. But I
mechanically pick up the needlework being offered me.

* * *

Every morning Dr. Schrock and Dr. Witek return to see
me. They somehow are my link with the sane world. Occasionally I feel a momentary flicker of hope—is there a
chance that somehow they can fix everything again?
But, they are for people with physical illnesses. Not for
people like me. I am depressed, neurotic, psychotic,
suicidal—there is nothing they can do for me now. But they
are kind—they really seem to care. I perceive the
psychiatrist as indifferent, cold, unfeeling. He just comes to
ask a few routine questions: "Are you going to group? Are
you suicidal?" He leaves as quickly as possible. I dread his
visits.
I am surrounded by other troubled souls. The ultimate in
pathos is a young Indian girl. Every morning she is wheeled
from the locked section dressed in pink footed pajamas,
thick ebony pigtails draped over her shoulders. An attendant parks her wheelchair directly across from the nurses'
station where she remains the entire day. She, too, is af-
flicted with a movement disorder. Her left arm is missing,
causing the pink sleeve to hang limply in her lap. She sits in
the same spot all day repeating the same word over and
over, sounding like "sah-rai...sah-rai...sah-rai." When a
nurse rations her one of two cigarettes for the day, she
stops. Her hand trembles as she brings the cigarette to her
mouth. She is quiet only until it's gone, then resumes her

unrelenting chant. Other patients try to distract her by coaxing her into looking at magazines. At the end of each day she disappears behind the locked doors.

For four days I am shoved from exercise group, to therapy, to OT, all of which I barely participate in. It is Friday. When the psychiatrist makes his daily stop he announces that I can leave tomorrow.

"I can't go home," I almost whisper. This place is no refuge, but there is none, and I can't go home again. Panic surges. Oh God, I don't want to stay here but I can't go home, either!

"Okay," the doctor responds dully. "You can go home Monday."

That's it. It is already decided. This man calls all the punches, orders my medication, arranges my daily schedule, tells me when to come and go. I don't like him. I don't trust him. But he is in control now. When you are crazy you need a shrink. But his guy couldn't care less about me or any of the other patients.

* * *

On Monday a stern-faced, heavyset nurse confronts me with a sheaf of papers in hand. She goes over a list of instructions, asking for my signature confirming that I understand them. I am to stay on all the medications and return to the psychiatrist in one month and Dr. Schrock in one week. After I sign them she looks at my face. "You still appear pretty anxious," she says, her tone accusing. "You have four kids and a husband at home. You just better pull yourself together, dear."

Oh God, if only she knew how badly I want to do just that!

*I cry to thee and thou dost
not hear me: I stand up,
and thou regardest me not*
Job 30:20

19

April 1985 - No escape

At home I continue to battle the extreme anxiety that fills
every moment of my conscious existence. My only escape is
the hypnotic drug, the tiny white pill, that takes me into
oblivion within minutes of swallowing it. The effects invariably last five hours, no more, no less. If I take it at 10
p.m., at exactly 3 a.m. I snap to as if I've been in a trance.
There's never any drowsiness or other sensation of having
slept. The only proof that any time has elapsed at all comes
from the alarm clock by my bed, whose hands have changed
positions.

For a long time I lie staring into the twilight. The bottles
of pills lined up on the table by my bed beckon constantly. If
I were to take all of them at once maybe they would wipe
everything out permanently. The ground outside is still
covered with snow. It must be below freezing. If I take the
pills first, then wander out to the park behind our property

and lie still in the snow, maybe no one will find me. They could go on then as if I'd never been a part of their lives. But what if Kim hears me get up, or Babe barks when I try to slip out the door? Someone might follow my footprints...

* * *

During the days I see the questioning fear in the children's eyes. There's nothing I can say to reassure them. Kim broke down and told them about the wrist-slashing, explaining that the drug was responsible. Jenny, Jason and Jonathan come and try to comfort me often. "It'll be okay Mom," they repeat as they put their arms around me. I know I love all of my family, that somewhere deep within my being the love will never go away. But I can't even feel the hugs through the terror.

Kim's sense of despair is apparent in his voice and actions. Once, as we stand face to face by the kitchen sink, he lifts his arm in the air as if to strike me, then lets it drop limply to his side. The look in his dark-lashed, grey-blue eyes is pleading, as if begging me to be well.

One day a friend stops by the house, tan from a trip to Hawaii with her husband. Amazingly, life is continuing around me. People are working, playing, laughing, in spite of my anguish. Oh God, I'm afraid for my family and my friends. If this horrible thing can happen to me, it can happen to any of them. Please don't let anyone else ever have to experience this kind of unconscionable fear.

Another dear friend comes to visit and pleads with tear-filled eyes to let her take me to the Mayo Clinic. "Please Linda, I've already told my boss that I'm going to take off work if you need me."

No escape

How can I explain that it doesn't matter now where I go.
That there's nothing they can do for me anymore.
Tomorrow is Easter. I struggle to keep things as normal
as possible. I remember tucking away some bags of candy in
my closet. I'm thankful that Kim's brother and his wife, Jim
and Jan, bring over some gifts for the children.
Kim is up before dawn. He goes alone to the sunrise service in the park, organized by three local churches. In spite
of his earlier denunciation of God, apparently he's gone back
to praying and seeking His help.
I manage to put together baskets of candy and the gifts
for the children. Our tradition has been to celebrate Easter
with my family at my house. This year Mom has invited
everyone to her home for dinner. Jerimiah drives the three
younger ones there for the day. Kim stays home with me.
Throughout the day he tries in vain to tame my tur-
bulence—talking, holding me, coaxing me to focus my attention on television. I can do nothing but pace like a caged
animal. Beside himself, exhausted from his efforts, Kim
finally informs me that he's decided to take me back to the
hospital in the city. This hospital is equipped for longer
term psychiatric patients and I can't face the other
psychiatrist. Kim's decision brings me no sense of relief.
In the morning according to plan, he leaves for the shop,
taking the two older boys to help. He will teach at the vocational school in the afternoon and by 7 p.m. will be back
home to take me to the hospital. Mid-morning Jenny and
Jonathan come to say good-bye before leaving for a friend's
house. Now I'm alone. It's better this way.
The bottles of pills are still lined up on the bedside table. I
despise them. I've taken them faithfully every day for two
weeks now—one week in the hospital and one at home, but

they're not helping me get well.

Water. I need a glass of water. I get up and go to the kitchen, filling a tall glass, then crawl back into bed. I won't stop now. It's just a matter of deciding which ones to take. Should I take all of them? The sleeping pills seem the most logical. They should work. Now that I know it's definite, I feel calmer. Picking up the small plastic bottle, I unscrew the cap and pour the contents in my palm. I count fourteen. I swallow them methodically, one by one, washing each down with a gulp of water. Should I continue and take all the other pills, too? For some reason I stop. Lying back down on the bed I wait, for what I don't know. I only know there can be no hell worse than the one I'm living in. Dear God, I was so sure of you. I trusted you. Please take care of Kim and the children. I know they will be better off without the burden of my craziness. At least they'll have a chance of living a normal life again.

* * *

I waken in a railed bed to the sound of a monitor beeping softly above my head. Intravenous tubes are taped to my arm. A clock on the wall to my left reads two o'clock. I gather from the dimness that it's two in the morning, not afternoon. When I am fully aware of myself, my muscles are jerking violently. The nightmare hasn't ended!

A petite, attractive young nurse with long, dark hair gets up from her station immediately outside of my door and comes to check on me. She has a worried look on her face. "I've been reading your chart. You've really been through a lot. I wish I could help you."

"How did I get here?"

No escape

"Your husband brought you in last night, about eight o'clock."

"I don't remember being brought here—I remember a stinging pain in my nose—shaking my head—nothing else."

"That was probably when they pumped your stomach. They inserted the tube down through your nose. Please, try to drink something." She holds a glass of water near my mouth.

"I can't," I protest, turning my head away. "I feel sick to my stomach."

The nurse goes back to her station. I watch the clock ticking away the minutes painfully slowly, convinced that time is in on a cruel hoax to keep me entrapped in my misery forever. I hear a voice coming from myself, crying, "God, please help me!"

When the clock hands finally creep their way to 6 a.m. a doctor arrives, introducing himself as the admitting physician from last night. After a brief appraisal of my condition, he announces that a psychiatrist will be in later. He picks up my chart as he leaves and then makes a phone call from the nursing station. I can hear part of the conversation—he's trying to reach Dr. Schrock.

The psychiatrist arrives after another eternity and orders tranquilizers. Then the dark-haired nurse comes back.

"Your mother-in-law phoned a little while ago. She said to tell you that she's coming to see you."

"No! Please tell her not to come. I don't want anyone to see me like this."

"It's too late. I'm sure she's on her way by now."

Oh God, she won't be able to understand that I am no longer part of their world. It isn't my choice, I'm just not. Just let me be alone in my misery, in my own black void.

LYME DISEASE: My Search for a Diagnosis

Somehow the clock has ticked away twelve hours. It is 2 p.m. now and they're going to move me to a new location. Mary is here with me as they unhook the wires and tubes and transfer me to a metal cart. She comes along as I'm wheeled down the hall into an elevator. Nobody has mentioned where they're taking me. They don't have to. As my cart is pushed up to the doors of the lock-up ward, panic and humiliation engulf me. I am gripping Mary's arm. "Don't put me in there. I can't go in there!"

The nurse ignores my cry and the doors are unlocked and opened. I am wheeled to a room beyond, one with a bed surrounded by stark white walls, nothing else. The only light is imbedded in the ceiling. A door leading to the bathroom is to be unlocked by a nurse when I need to use it. My clothing and purse that Kim brought the night before are removed.

"You'll probably be staying here for a few days. We'll just have you stay in your pajamas. Dr. Steele, a neurologist, will come up to check you."

Dr. Steele. Am I hearing her right? Is it the same Dr. Steele I doctored with for the first two years of my illness, who was convinced I was neurotic from the start? I didn't know he was on staff here. It is painfully ironic that he should be the one to see me like this. I had prayed for so long that he would believe that I was mentally sound. This fits the living nightmare perfectly.

It is the same Dr. Steele. He is looming over my bed with a half-smile on his face. "Linda and I have known each other for quite awhile," he remarks to the nurse.

"I guess you've been right all these years. I am crazy." I don't see any purpose in the exam. I don't need a neurologist. But Dr. Steele is proceeding anyway.

"Let's see you run your heel down your shin."

- 120 -

No escape

I do as I'm told, but I'm wishing he'd go away, I wish they'd all go away. I don't want Mary telling me everything is going to be all right when it's not.

"I want you to try to stand up," Dr. Steele says.

I try, but fall to my knees.

"After what you did to yourself, it's going to take a little time."

He's finally gone. Later in the evening, after Mary leaves, two nurses return with a wheelchair. "We're going to move you to a different room."

"I thought you said that I was going to stay here for a few days," I say timidly, glancing up in time to catch a wink between the two of them. They don't answer. Why are they doing this? Can I trust them?

My new room is a few doors away. It has a closet and a night stand. The bathroom door is unlocked. One of the nurses retrieves my clothing and hangs it in the closet. They leave my door open and a patient from the adjoining room comes to pay a visit. She stands in the doorway, only one foot inside the room. She's obese, probably in her thirties, with thick, wavy, jet black hair. Too much make-up creates a clown-like image—a rather ominous looking figure. Her language tops her appearance for repugnance. In a raspy whisper she begins telling me of her many past sexual encounters.

"You know, I could have been a movie star," she hisses. She goes on, informing me of the evilness of the hospital staff, of vile things they do to patients here where no one will know and no one will believe us if we tell them. "You better be ready. They'll be in here tonight. I'll give you some advice. Just hold your breath till you pass out. That's the only way you'll be able to stand it."

LYME DISEASE: My Search for a Diagnosis

I gawk at her, not daring to respond. It turns out to be only the first of several informative visits from her that evening.

Mom comes and stays for awhile, trying to console me. When she leaves I crawl to the corner of my room and huddle against the register like a cornered mouse with no place to hide. The nurses return and attempt to assure me that there's nothing to be afraid of, that the clown woman is harmless. Who can I believe?

I sit up all night clutching the bed sheet over me, rankled by terrifying images of wicked people doing vile things to me, the clown woman smothering me with her massive form. All the vileness of the world seems to parade through my brain. Will this be the final cut-off between Kim and me and our family and friends? Will they finally flee in disgust as far as they can from me?

Eventually the night breaks through to morning. No one has come to my room except to do bed checks. I'm beginning to realize that the hospital staff sincerely wants to help me. I'm still weak when I try to stand. A nurse brings me out into the main room in a wheelchair, where we are greeted by the noisy clanking of breakfast trays. Patients are picking up meals and assembling around a long Formica table to eat. Most of them have the same vacant expression on their faces; a few are muttering to themselves. The clown woman, her bulging eyes still heavily rimmed with black mascara, dark rouge circling her cheeks, is babbling incessantly to anyone within hearing about her grandiose experiences, punctuating her narration with bouts of cursing.

Setting a breakfast in front of me, the nurse leaves me next to the table with a half dozen other patients. I see no purpose in putting nourishment into this pathetic body that has become only a holding place for my tormented spirit—a spirit that seems doomed to exist no matter how fervently I want it to die.

The morning becomes a blur of doctors and other people coming and going. Mom and Mary return and are here when Dr. Steele stops by again. He mentions something about sending me to the Mayo Clinic. I'm surprised that he is bringing this up now. I'm too brittle to go anywhere.

In the afternoon I sit frozen in a chair observing the other patients. A distraught looking young man dressed in hospital pajamas walks up to the nurses' station and begins explaining to the attendants that he wasn't always deranged. His hair juts out in matted tufts. I too feel a compulsion to make the attendants understand that I was a part of their sane world once, but they'll never understand—and how can it possibly make any difference to them?

I loathe the fact that I'm here, that I've become what I've become, but nothing can change what has happened. I have a sickening awareness that this is where I belong.

Later I look up to see the security guard unlocking the doors of the ward to allow someone to enter. When I realize that it's Kim I feel a fleeting glimmer of hope. That he still wants anything to do with me is astounding. He looks handsome in his casual tan slacks and sweater. He quickly scans the ward, then fixes his eyes on me as I get up to meet him. They no longer reflect anger, only a deep sadness and futility.

If there were only some way I could put our lives back in order. We're both at a loss for words. What can we possibly say? No words can soothe the pain. I need to know that the kids are okay. My four beautiful, healthy, loving children. How can they survive knowing that their mother is mad?

My attempts to remove myself from their lives have failed. Lord, if I have to endure this agony, why can't you at least allow me to be removed far enough away that they won't have to know it and be a part of it?

Kim seems uneasy about being here. His eyes dart nervously. He tries to sound matter-of-fact, but he's talking quickly, clenching and unclenching his fists. He doesn't stay long, mentioning something about meeting a customer concerning an upcoming job.

By my second day in the ward I am no longer afraid of any of the other patients, even the clown woman. I overhear some of the attendants saying she will soon be on her way to a more permanent place. Is that going to by my fate, too? I know I can't stay here forever. Where else can I possibly go?

A nurse is telling me they want to move me out of this section to the "free" area of the psych ward. "Can you make a pact with me that you won't try to hurt yourself?" she asks.

I look into her impassive face and wonder what she will do if I say no? I don't know what I'll do; I don't trust myself. My bizarre, intense anxiety has calmed somewhat to a haunting depression that feels no better to me, but somehow my outward demeanor has deceived them into believing I'm doing better. It doesn't make any difference; I might as well say what they want to hear. I nod affirmatively. The nurse leaves to make arrangements for me to be moved.

My anxiety about leaving the lock-up section makes the move almost as traumatic as entering. As revolted as I am by this place, in the few days I've been here I've formed a distasteful sort of attachment, a sense of belonging. The "free" section is new, uncertain, even more frightening.

My new room is near the nurses' station. A big "C5"

No escape

backgrounded by a yellow square on the wall next to the station labels the floor and the section. Esther, my new roommate, is a shadow of a woman in her eighties, her white hair wisping around her lined face. She listens to a Christian radio station, crochets, and colors pictures with a pack of child's crayons. "Just to make the time pass," she explains in a crackling voice.

She tells me that her husband is in another hospital, that they didn't want them to be in the same place. "Listening to Christian radio programs used to help, but it doesn't now. I always read the Bible regularly, but my eyesight isn't so good anymore," she adds, picking up her Bible and paging through it. "Maybe if I had someone who could read it to me..."

"I'll read to you," I offer. I begin with the chapter that she has marked in Psalms, praying that some meaning will come through the words for Esther and for me. But there's nothing. The words seem hollow and meaningless, unable to penetrate my barrier of fear. When I finish, Esther shakes her head sadly. "I always found comfort in the Bible before; I don't know why it's not working," she says.

I desperately want to feel normal again, to find my way out of this pit, to regain my shattered faith. I think of the teens in my Sunday school class. A month ago I was moved by their sincerity and their eagerness to learn more about God. I had actually believed that I had something to give them. They had looked up to me and now at the very least I've let them down, maybe destroyed their faith.

I listened to Jonathan say his prayers one night before I came here. With tears brimming in his eyes, he had said, "Please God, don't let my mom have to go back in the hospital."

Oh God, I tried not to.

And Kim, who rarely talked about his faith, though I knew it was there—deeper, more sincere than many who are more vocal—what has this done to his faith? I am tormented by these thoughts.

Eventually I will come to realize that every person's faith is his own gift from God, that I couldn't take it away anymore than I could give it.

In spite of my sense of futility, I continue to read to Esther from her Bible, and I ask Kim to bring me one from home.

20

Late April 1985 - Never-ending fear

"When I consider him I am afraid of him" Job 23:15.

Winter's grasp is failing—the snow has melted, the trees in the park are budding, and grass is beginning to revive. The weather has warmed enough that others have shed winter coats for light jackets and sweaters, but I'm still wearing my tan quilted coat. For me there is no sense of spring's renewal, only a hazy greyness, flat and colorless.

As my feet plod mechanically along the sidewalk, I am barely aware of the other bodies and faces passing me. I try focusing my attention on the external world to distract myself from my own pall of gloom. Some of the faces belong to young men and women carrying books, probably students from the nearby college. I see them only as a taunting reminder of my shattered hope to someday go back to school, maybe even get my college degree. Was it possible that once I was really that confident in myself?

Glancing up, I accidentally meet the gaze of an old man, cane in hand, limping along on the other side of the walk. He nods at me, his weathered face crinkling into a smile. I go through the motions of responding, straining the corners of my mouth into a mock smile. To him I probably look no different than others strolling by.

I am different, though. They are sane, capable, functioning human beings; I am not. Perhaps the only visible distinction is the hospital band fastened to my wrist. I'm feeling the same concrete under my feet, breathing the same air, hearing the same city traffic sounds. Yet I'm separate from it, trapped in my own impenetrable, dark world.

How many times have I circled the park now? Has any time passed at all? Time. It persists in inching its way along almost imperceptibly. The only purpose in my motion is somehow to make time pass. Once across from the hospital again, I turn and aim myself in the direction of the brick and concrete structure looming coldly in front of me. Should I go back in? It doesn't make any difference. Sooner or later I'll have to. There is nowhere else to go.

I wait for the traffic to wane, then move in the direction of the building. I push through the glass doors, past the stained glass mural, take a right and approach a second set of doors that slide open automatically. I've passed the attendants at the reception desk and information center dozens of times in the weeks I've been here without ever seeing their faces. Moving toward the square labeled C Building, I take one left turn, then another, and face a row of elevator doors interrupting a sky blue wall. I press the up arrow.

The elevator jolts to a stop and the doors open on C5. I

walk straight ahead to the desk and sign in, glancing at the clock. Only about twenty minutes overcome. Still three more hours until dinnertime. The nurses at the station are going about their business and don't bother to look up as I fill in my name and time of return. A few patients sit in the lounge area watching TV. Television makes me even more edgy.

A plain-looking young nurse walks towards me. "Linda, why didn't you go to group today?"

"I-I can't sit through it any more. I've tried. It's just not helping me. I get nothing out of it."

Her voice reflects her annoyance. "Well, if you don't take advantage of what we have to offer, how can you expect to be helped?"

"Fine, I'll go back tomorrow," I respond flatly.

I don't tell her about my aversion to Tammy, one of the group leaders. She makes the almost two-hour afternoon sessions even more unbearable. Tammy had interviewed me to determine which group I would be placed in. "Tell me what kind of problems you had prior to coming here," she had demanded. I repeated that there were no problems except for the strange, nameless illness that has plagued me for four years. Everything else in my life was fine, including my relationship with my husband, children, friends, and work. And I was coping fairly well with the illness until after I'd started the Prednisone. I could think of nothing that would bring me to the mental state I am in.

"Well, obviously you're denying something," she shot back with cocky sureness. She seemed to enjoy her power over me. I was dismayed to discover she had assigned me to her own group.

Tammy sits slouching lazily in her chair, slurping on a can

of Coke. Her superior air seems intended to let me know that she knows more about me than I know about myself. The sessions seem filled with pointless banter, punctuated with crude language. When Tammy and the group members urge me to pour out my problems I can think of nothing to say. I won't mention the illness again. Every time I do someone writes in my chart that I'm preoccupied with physical symptoms. They want me to talk about my *real* problems. According to them, if no one has been able to diagnose the cause of my bizarre symptoms after this long, they must be psychological. "You're denying something," I am told over and over till it echoes in my head. What am I denying? When I beg them to help me, they can offer no clues.

The nurse leaves and I pick up the phone to dial Mom's number. If I don't call her I know she'll call anyway and make idle conversation—trying to think of humorous incidents to lighten my mood. But there is no lightness, no humor in my dismal world.

My chorea movement, less obvious for the past several days, has started up again. At first some of the other patients were unnerved by my odd contortions. Marge, a young girl who complains of out-of-body experiences, screamed the first time she saw them. She went running to fetch a nurse before I could stop her. Yet, with the chorea active I'm more readily accepted by the patients. I have a tangible problem, a reason for being here.

When it's finally dinnertime I wait in line for my tray. I've been able to get food down, although I don't care whether I do or not. I eat in case there's the slightest chance that something in the food chemistry can restore a balance in my system. Somewhere I read that nutritional deficiencies can cause mental disorders.

Never-ending fear

Steve and Bob are already in the cafeteria and nod as I sit down across the table from them. The other patients shuffle in one at a time. There is a sort of grim comaraderie among the inmates here. Even the most sardonic reach out of themselves on occasion to offer some meager comfort to the other troubled souls inhabiting the ward. Our sickness has become our common bond. Everyone here has come to the point where we are unable to cope with life. Most have attempted, or at least have considered, suicide as a way of escape. We are all barely existing. I have gotten plenty of advice from these fellow patients in the weeks I've been here.

Steve is an institutional veteran, already on his fourteenth hospital stay in his attempt to overcome alcohol addiction. His solid physique belies what medical tests have revealed—his drinking has taken its toll systemically. His ever-present hand tremors betray his insecurity. This time, he says, he will make it after leaving here. He has lectured and counseled me. "You're responsible for pulling yourself up by your own bootstraps." He talks confidently, yet he hasn't been able to pull things together to work for himself.

Bob, small-framed and neatly groomed, comes across as tough and steely, even surly at times. Before coming here he drove himself hard, working three jobs to support his family. Now his wife has taken his children away and is asking for a divorce. He was brought to a holding room one night by the police after he threatened to jump from a bridge. When he learned that my first suicide attempt involved slashing my wrists he explained that I'd gone about it all wrong and gave me carefully detailed instructions on the proper way to do it. In spite of his cynical attitude I don't dislike him.

Shirley is the most negative person I've ever encountered. Only in her twenties, she has a haggard look. She grew up with an abusive father, has struggled with severe depression all her life, and is certain that life has no meaning. For her, God has never existed and she responds bitterly to anyone who suggests otherwise. Yet, even she, during my worst moments, attempts to reassure me that things will get better.

Occasionally another patient is released. I'm disturbed that so many of them return home only to be readmitted a short time later. Ann is back after being out only a week. She's started shock treatments again. In a continual trance-like state, she makes no attempt to communicate even with other patients and leaves her room only at mealtimes.

Dick, a meek man who reminds me of my dad, also went through a series of shock treatments, which helped only temporarily. A former professor with big plans to travel, he was forced into premature retirement by his unexpected depression. He has confided to me that his only prayer each night is that he'll die during his sleep. Everything seems so hopeless. Doesn't anyone around here get well and stay that way?

Two other patients on the ward are convinced that prescribed drugs have brought them to their present state. I balk at taking more medication because I, too, believe it was the drug that caused my problem in the first place. But I can't survive without tranquilizers and the hospital staff has persisted until I've agreed to try a low dose of an anti-depressant.

After dinner I retreat to my room, alone, with more endless hours to kill before another long, sleepless night. Kim won't be coming this evening. He tries to get here as often as possible, a couple of evenings a week and Saturday or Sunday. He brings the children on weekends, but never allows them to come up to the fifth floor. They wait downstairs in the lobby. I meet them there and sometimes we go for an outing. Yesterday was Jerimiah's seventeenth birthday. We all went out to dinner to celebrate. I managed to save my morning tranquilizer and take two before we left. Jerimiah, always thoughtful, bought me two books written by Christian authors. "I know that you like this kind of book, Mom," he had said. On *his* birthday he brought *me* gifts.

The family visits are important to me. I need to see they are okay even though I feel that I'm failing them and am terribly unworthy of their love.

I'm glad that our friends heed Kim's advice not to come here. It's hard enough when relatives stop by—Mom and Dad, Mary and Bob, and my brothers, Jim and John. My belief that I'll never live up to their expectations that I can recover from this madness makes it agonizing to see them. I'm almost certain that a permanent residence in a mental institution is inevitable. Still I can't bring myself to tell anyone. I'll spare them as long as possible.

I have no idea who or what is the author of this state of chaotic terror that my life has become. Is it the illness, the Prednisone, or am I the enemy, the originator of my own ruin? Deep down I still can't believe that I am, but how can I fight it? How can I plead my case when it's clear that I'm mentally unstable?

I keep praying to my God, yet He remains fearsome and elusive. My cries are met with silence, no answers come. I can't deny God's existence or the time in my life when I felt His love so acutely it was as though He had reached out and touched me. Has He turned on me, become sadistic? Or has this pit separated me so far from Him that He can't even hear my cries? I recite 2 Timothy 1:7 over and over in my mind, as I have so many times in the past years. *God hath not given us a spirit of fear, but of power and of love and of a sound mind.* I remain desperately afraid—helpless, rejected and confused.

I remind myself that God has pulled me out of dark places before and restored my faith. But this pit is bottomless, so much blacker than any I've encountered before. Voices from the unidentifiable enemy are continually shouting through the darkness that there is no way out of this one. I try to shut them out. I strain to hear another, faint, barely distinguishable voice that insists the faith that I had was real. That no matter how hopeless everything appears, there might be a way out. I can't give up—not yet.

21

Late April 1985 continued - Going home

When I am told by my doctors that eighty percent of those suffering from clinical depression get well, all I hear is that twenty percent don't. Somebody has to be part of the twenty percent and I fear that I am one of them.

"You're getting better," Dr. Adams, the bearded psychiatrist, keeps telling me. "You seem much less intense."

I don't believe him. It's impossible for me to see the positive side of anything. But that doesn't stop me from trying. I pick out Bible verses and some days I recite the same one over and over in my mind. I practice positive self-talk. I'm told that guilt will hinder a depressed person's recovery. If I have been fabricating my illness all these years, then I am guilty of causing my friends and family a great deal of distress. But I didn't scheme it. I struggle not to submit to the feelings of guilt. If I do, then every ounce of hope will be lost. When the guilt tries to overpower me I continually renounce it.

I know that inevitably the subject of my release will come up. Finally Dr. Adams tells me that it is time to start thinking about going home. I dread it. The sooner I go home, the sooner everyone will realize that I can't make it in the real world anymore. I can never belong. Then there will be the awfulness of Kim and the children knowing what I already know.

"What are you going to do about your job?" Dr. Adams asks one day.

"I don't know...I don't think I can go back."

"Why not? Can't you just plan to go back part time?"

The idea of going back at all seems incomprehensible. Yet I can't bear the thought of making Kim drag home all my shelves, machines, and fabric when he'd worked so hard to help me set it up.

"Why don't we plan on Thursday for your discharge date?" Dr. Adams is saying.

Oh God, I'm scared. I had hoped to be able at least to learn how to sleep again before being discharged. Sleep has eluded me for so long I am convinced that whatever part of my brain controls it has ceased to function. I am determined not to ask for sleeping pills, but every hour of every night I meet with open eyes the blinding glare of the flashlight carried by the attendant doing bed check. I postpone bed times as long as possible hoping that exhaustion will eventually win out.

On a typical night, no earlier than eleven o'clock, I pull a pair of hospital pajamas from the linen cupboard in the lobby, head down to the cafeteria and warm a glass of milk in the microwave. The nurse offers me relaxation tapes with

Going home

droning voices and sounds of ocean waves, designed to relieve tension. I take my nightly ration of medication and try to read from the Bible Kim brought. But I still don't sleep. I'm up checking the hall clock. Two, three, four a.m. go by. Finally I fall into a restless semi-sleep for an hour or two before dawn. I'm wide awake again before 7 a.m. when Kim calls from his shop. He calls faithfully every day announcing that everything is "fine" at home. I know that it's not really fine. How can it be? They must all be suffering a great deal, too.

* * *

Kim comes to pick me up on May third, almost four weeks from my admission date. Later on as I look back, I will see that my mental state is much improved from when I was released from the other hospital the previous month. But now I am too blinded by my own fears to see it. My shattered ego has me believing that I will never again be a respectable wife and mother.

Kim knows I am extremely apprehensive. "The kids are really looking forward to having you home," he offers. I wish I could say I am looking forward to being home, too.

When I entered the hospital, winter had been lingering, but now spring has fully unfolded. Bright tulips and daffodils, border yards. People are starting to till gardens to get them ready for planting. Patches of black dirt await new seeds.

As Kim pulls the car up to our back door, I spot Jenny and Jonathan. Perched on top of the white picket fence, Jonathan jumps off and joins his sister, who is running toward us shouting excitedly, "Mom's home! Mom's home!'' I am almost thrown off balance by the weight of their bodies plowing into me, engulfing me with hugs. Jerimiah and Jason are putting down rakes and heading across the yard at a fast clip. Although more reserved, they too give me hugs and their delight at having me back home is obvious in their dancing eyes. My certainty that I am only going to disappoint them destroys my ability to share the joy they are expressing. Somehow I have to hide my fear from them.

Kim announces his intention to be barbecue chef and goes to start the grill. "We'll go to the grocery store to pick up some pork chops to throw on for supper," he says. While I'd been gone they all survived on frozen pizzas, frozen chicken, canned soup and tuna fish sandwiches. Kim had stubbornly refused to take any more help from friends and relatives. When people called he always said, "We're doing fine. Just pray for Linda."

We tell the children we'll be back soon and climb back into the car. I am apprehensive. What if I run into someone I know? What if I panic? But as we pass by the familiar sights—the city park, the corner grocery market, the cafes, the beauty shop, our sewing shop—buildings that had been part of my life for so many years, a tiny glimmer of light comes. Maybe, just maybe, I will someday belong here again, to this little town that houses my children's schools, provided a place to start a business, and places to run errands and attend community functions.

"I'll wait for you in the car," I tell Kim as he stops in front of the grocery store. I wait anxiously for him to return, frantically hoping I won't see any familiar faces. In a few minutes Kim returns, plunking the brown paper sack into the back seat.

Going home

The grill is ready by the time we get back. "I'll take care of the pork chops and you can do the potatoes and salad," he directs.

I unload the groceries and wash the potatoes and vegetables for our salad. I am functioning but not functioning. It's a facade that will come crumbling down at any moment. I am just going through motions. How long can I keep it up? Five minutes? An hour? A day? Then it will be helter skelter again, a jumbled boundless nightmare.

The children are chatting happily as we sit down to the kitchen table. They've accepted me back with no questions, simply content that I'm here. I don't know how much Jenny and Jonathan know about what happened or if they understand where I've been. I wish I could protect them.

"Mom, guess what? I've learned how to wash the floor now," Jenny proudly announces. "I used the sponge mop, the one you never use."

Jason is enthusiastic about an MS bike-a-thon he's been planning to participate in and shares information about it.

They all seem so grown up. Jenny is eleven already and starting to mature. Jerimiah has begun shaving. Jason, at fifteen, has finally passed me in height. Even Jonathan, with his cherub face, is looking more adult.

When dinner is over I start clearing the table. I can tell that the effect of the Xanax (the tranquilizer) is wearing off. Dr. Adams keeps telling me I need to take them on a regular basis. But I fight taking them. I don't want to become addicted. It bothers me that I need a higher dose to have an effect than when I first started them. I have gone from the 25mg white tablets to the 50mg peach ones. Twice the dosage, and they no longer make me groggy. It means that I'm building up a tolerance for them. What if I need to go to yet a higher dose? One of the other patients in the hospital claimed to have become addicted to Valium prescribed for back problems. In the hospital she had spent all day pacing, crying, walking half-doubled over and shaking. They put her on three new medications. It was an endless vicious cycle of drugs.

How badly I want not to be dependent on pills, but I am. As much as I hate them, the idea of leaving the house without having them in my purse leaves me shaking inside.

The children are heading for the TV room, while Kim stays to help clean up the kitchen. "I've made up my mind that I'm going to take some time off this summer and we'll do some fun things with the kids," he announces. "What would you like to do?"

Why is he asking me? Please don't make me make decisions. It's too overwhelming. I don't know if I can make it through the next ten minutes, let alone plan days and weeks ahead.

"I...I don't know...you decide."

For years I had tried to convince Kim to take more time off work to do more family things and now that he is doing it I can't even get excited.

"I thought we could go tubing down the Apple River one day, maybe drive down to Rochester for a few days and stay in a hotel, go to the Omni Theatre," he goes on.

"That would be really nice," I say, trying to sound sincere. I can see that I haven't fooled him, though. His face reveals disappointment that I'm not showing more enthusiasm.

"Tomorrow, we'll need to go grocery shopping when I get home from work. I talked to Maxine this morning and she said just to let her know when you're ready to go back to work."

Going home

Oh God. I can't understand how they can continue to believe in my ability to function. How am I going to tell them that I can't go back? Yet the thought of staying home is equally unsettling.

I make no response and Kim is furrowing his thick dark brows. "You are going back, aren't you?"

"I'll try."

I feel like I'm standing in quicksand and will begin sinking any moment. I know I won't make it. My being home is only temporary. Next time I go away, it won't be for a short stay. I'll be locked up somewhere for good.

My heart is in turmoil,
and is never still; days of
affliction come to meet me
Job 30:27 RSV

22

Mid June 1985 - Functioning but not functioning

Physically I am doing better than I have in years. Only a few symptoms remain and they are mild. The chorea has subsided. Outwardly our lives seem on an even keel. The children are happily occupied with summer jobs and activities. We have followed through on some of the planned family excursions.

At work now I am finishing the faces of the kittens I've appliqued on the dresses and sweatsuits I made today. It's been over a month since I returned to the shop, but I'm still unbelieving. At one time I would have been pleased with my creations. But my certainty that my sanity isn't here to stay continues to overshadow my ability to feel any positive emotion.

Maxine is talking on the phone and now her hearty laughter fills the room. The ability to laugh—that must be the secret of wellness. I can't remember the last time I laughed. Why am I different? How can other people laugh while I feel no trace of joy?

I've been staying busy. In fact if physical exertion and keeping busy are a panacea for depression, I should be getting better. I have planted the garden and gotten the house back in order. I'm working at the shop three days a week. I'm deeply afraid of having any idle time or time alone.

Mondays are the worst. We close our shop that day. Kim is at work, and if the kids are visiting friends I might be home alone. I invite friends over for coffee.

"You look really good," they keep telling me. I wonder how long I can fool them into thinking I'm okay. They don't know that every second of every day is a battle to keep the anxiety at a manageable level—a battle to go one extra hour without taking the Xanax. Dr. Adams insisted that I stay on the antidepressant, too. I'm convinced it's not helping, but I take it to appease him. Time is still my constant enemy; I can't believe that once it moved faster than I wanted it to. Now every day seems to drag endlessly, no matter how many activities are planned. The thought of getting through weeks, months, and years feels awesome. I start marking days off on the calendar, just so I can look at it and prove to myself time is passing. But whenever I look at it, I only see too many more days ahead to conquer.

Maxine hangs up the phone, chuckling to herself now. She comes over to inspect my projects. "Those are really cute. I should have you make a dress for my granddaughter. And just think, you thought you wouldn't be able to come back to work. I'm really proud that you're doing so well! How did your appointment in Buffalo go?"

"Okay," I lie. As usual I had come out of the psychologist's office feeling worse than when I went in. A friend had recommended him as a Christian counselor. It isn't that I don't think he's trying, but we're getting nowhere. I'm searching for some indication that God still cares, but if He's around He's being extremely elusive. I need to stop reliving the past, but I don't know how. I am plagued with questions that no one can answer. The psychologist asked if I thought God had caused my problems. I don't believe that He caused them but I know He allowed them. I can't stop believing that it's just chance that I'm still alive. I learned later that if I'd taken the whole bottle of antidepressants instead of the sleeping pills I wouldn't have survived. The psychologist suggested that the fact that my life was spared is evidence that God had been watching over me, but I can't believe that either. Sometimes I am sent home from appointments with books about positive thinking and positive self-talk. I can find no meaning in them. I've already tried all the tricks and gimmicks. They haven't worked. The books sound so simple—written for people with low self-esteem. At one time I believe I had a reasonably good self-image. It didn't help me. In fact I used positive self-talk and prayer right through the suicide attempts. They just didn't work.

I am still seeing Dr. Adams once a month to manage my medication. He always asks the same superficial questions and offers the same advice. What are you doing to stay busy? How's your husband's business? Try to be less intense. Try not to think so hard. Take the medication on a regular basis.

Maxine is engrossed in her own work now. According to the wall clock it is almost closing time. I gather up my scraps from the cutting table and throw them in the waste basket, unplug my iron, and hang the garments on hangers.

Why can't I feel good about the accomplishments? I've made it through another whole day at work. I only see it as being one day closer to the day I break down, lose the struggle and go sliding back into the pit. Only the tranquilizers keep me going at all. One day they'll lose their effectiveness. I skipped taking two today, but maybe tomorrow I'll need more.

23

August 1985 - An endless tunnel

I have the same sinking feeling after today's church service that I've had every Sunday since I came home from the hospital. But I keep coming back, praying that something in the Scripture reading, the music, the sermon will provide consolation or inspiration.

I am heading down the gold and brown carpeted steps to our church basement asking myself why I am bothering to stay for the Bible study. I know if I go home I won't feel any better. I seem to keep walking through an endless tunnel and no matter how far I go I'm not seeing a light at the end.

I keep hoping something will click to rekindle my faith. Whatever is left of it is so fragile it's almost nonexistent. I refuse to let go of the fragment. It's like hanging on to a twig to keep from sliding over the edge of a steep cliff. Still I'm clinging with every ounce of strength I have even though my sense of reason tells me it's no use. It'll never be strong enough to pull me back up.

The tables are pushed together to form a U-shape with the chairs arranged around the edge. Almost all of the seats are occupied. I spot an empty chair next to Jean and walk past the other people towards it. The discussion is already underway. I open my study book to the page that I see Jean reading from and try to absorb the information being related. They are studying the Old Testament. The sermons lately have been based on the Old Testament, too. All they talk about is killing, plagues, and suffering. I can find nothing uplifting in it. It only makes me more depressed. As usual I wind up tuning out most of the conversation.

When it's over, everyone gets up and leaves, except Jean. For some reason we're both stalling. She turns to me and smiles. "Linda, I'm glad you're here. I've been meaning to ask you how things are going."

I try to answer, but my words are choked back with sobs.

"How would you like to come over to my house and talk?" she offers kindly. "I'm free any time this afternoon or evening."

I nod, trying to regain my composure.

"What time do you want to come?"

"It...doesn't matter...Anytime!" I manage to blurt.

"Let's make it right after supper. About seven?"

"Okay."

She gives me a squeeze. "Good, I'll see you later then."

I cry all the way home. For those weeks I was in the hospital I hadn't been able to cry at all. Now the tears are triggered too easily and are hard to stop.

Kim is relieved that I'm going to talk to Jean. She's a trained counselor and he's always had a high opinion of her.

An endless tunnel

Kim is one of the few who is still aware of my continuing inner conflict. He knows how fragile my psyche really is.

Jean's house is nestled in a woods at the end of a long winding driveway. She offers me a glass of lemonade and ushers me to a cozy room with rows of windows on three sides, where it's possible to view a good share of the surrounding wooded yard. Here we're alone, but not isolated from the world.

I explain to Jean my need to know that there is some purpose in the whole mess. Somehow I know I'll never be okay unless I can put my experience behind me, and I know I can't do it without God's help. I don't understand how people who claim to be agnostic or atheists can face the hopelessness their stated beliefs imply. I know that without faith I can't survive.

With Jean's encouragement I spill my guts, telling her everything that happened before and after the Prednisone. I tell her about my guilt and self-doubt—the years of questioning whether or not my illness is real or psychological and all the gory details of the suicide attempts and my stays in the hospital. By the varying expressions on her face I see that Jean is reliving my ordeal along with me. When I finish she shares her own feelings.

"Wow, Linda, that's really awful!" she says empathetically. "You have a right to be angry and frightened. In fact, right now I'm feeling pretty angry at God myself!"

While I was in the hospital, one nurse had tried to get me to express anger toward God, but I found it impossible to vent an emotion I didn't feel; I only felt a great fear and uncertainty.

I feel accepted by Jean and soothed by her manner. That she seems to agree that my feelings are appropriate for what

I've been through is important to me. She doesn't ask why, as so many others have done. I can never answer that. I don't know why I am the way I am. I just am. Her unaccusing, unquestioning empathy hints at the beginning of a healing process. Having Jean walk back through the entire nightmare with me has lightened the load just enough to make it a fraction more bearable. There has been no one else that I've dared share as much with. Everyone else wants to gloss it over, pretend it hasn't happened. "Just go on, Linda. Everything will be fine." Jean doesn't try to simplify the problem with superficial phrases.

"If you want, Linda, I'm willing to have you come back and talk on a weekly basis. I could set aside one evening a week. I'm not involved in any particular Christian service right now and I've been praying that God would show me what I could do. Maybe your sitting next to me in Bible study wasn't an accident?"

"If you have the time, then yes, I'd really like that."

Our talk has already stretched close to two and a half hours and I know I must leave now. I'm glad I'll be coming back next Thursday. The shadows from the trees are lengthening as I pull my car out of the driveway. I'm afraid to hope, yet afraid not to hope that somehow Jean can help guide me out of this maze of despair and confusion that has woven itself into every thread of my being.

24

Fall 1985 · A glimmer of light

Jean's home and her patient, listening ear have become my haven. One thing Jean seems to have is a sense of purpose, organization, a plan. We structure our sessions around a series of contracts. I promise I will tell her or someone else if I begin feeling suicidal and we agree to meet on a regular basis for four months. We will then evaluate the situation with input from Kim. After our first meeting she asks me to go home and make lists of things about which I feel sad, happy, angry, ashamed, and afraid. I have difficulty thinking of anything to put on most of the lists. I stare at the blank pages, which in a former time would have been easy to fill. But those emotions no longer exist for me. Only my fear list I could write endlessly, starting with "getting up in the morning." From there I add "going to work, not going to work, being alone, facing people, life, death, time, God..."

Jean's faith is strong. Mine is almost nonexistent. I often

think about the Bible verse that promises that if your faith
is as small as a mustard seed you will be able to move moun-
tains. I am sure mine is smaller than that.

Our weekly sessions have continued through August,
September, October. Most of our visits stretch close to two
hours and it is always with reluctance that I decide I've
taken up enough of her time.

With Jean I have replayed my early years, dredging up
every negative life experience I can recall. If there is really
something subconscious that I'm denying that's keeping
me from getting well, I'm determined to figure out what it
is.

As a child I had low self-esteem and was so shy that some
of my teachers were worried. At times I overheard them
talking about me in the hallway. My sixth grade teacher
kept me in from recess more than once asking questions
about my home life, trying to determine why I was so timid.

My mother was stern and yelled a lot, except when I was
sick. Then she softened and I really felt that she cared about
me. It has occurred to me a number of times during my illness that maybe subconsciously I believed that I need to be
sick to be loved. Yet I wasn't a sickly child, other than occasional tonsillitis and flu—typical childhood illnesses. As an
adult I've had a satisfying relationship with my mom and
am confident of her love.

Meeting Kim was a major turning point in my life. As our
relationship deepened, my feelings of self worth grew. Kim
and I were engaged at seventeen and married two years
later. Maybe we'd still had some growing up to do, but
we've never been sorry and both value our marriage and
family.

According to our own observations and those of other
family members, friends, and school teachers, all of our

children are well adjusted and loving. It is difficult for me to believe that they could be flourishing so well if their mother were severely disturbed all these years.

At the end of our sessions Jean prays with me. I am comforted. I feel that her faith is carrying us both. My own prayers seem so futile.

Jean has asked me to keep lists each day rating my mood on a scale of one to ten. One is really a bad day, ten a super day. All my days remain between one and three. Between sessions I continue to do everything I can to distract myself from the cloud of gloom that hovers around me.

All four of the children are playing on various softball teams this summer. The games we attend almost every evening have become one of my few escapes. When I watch, I find I can tune out almost everything else. As another mental distraction I have started looking through the dictionary picking out words and learning definitions to try to keep my mind occupied. But these diversions aren't solving the problem. I remain dependent on tranquilizers to get through the days and to sleep at night which creates its own dilemma. I still worry that I'll become addicted to the pills that provide relief. By now the main thrust of my praying is that, for my family's sake, I'll die a less shameful death before I'm driven to suicide again or am locked away somewhere.

* * *

Today Ken, a friend and former member of our church, stopped by and left a cassette tape for me. He said that it contains a sermon presented by the minister of his current church. When he's gone I pick it up and read the title, "Going Through a Test—I Corinthians 10:13." That verse is one that I memorized in a Bible study I attended prior to the Prednisone. It had come back to me a number of times during my ordeal. As I know it in the King James version it says, "There hath no temptation taken you, but such as is common to man; but God is faithful, who will not suffer you to be tempted beyond what you are able, but will with the temptation also provide a way of escape that you may be able to bear it." That verse brings no comfort. Instead I react with anger. My impulse is to throw the cassette across the room. I despair that there's nothing in it that will help me. If I listen to it I'll probably just feel worse than I already do. But Ken is a friend; he's trying to help. Reluctantly I slip the tape into the recorder.

In spite of my resistance the narrator captures my attention almost immediately. I am intrigued by Pastor Dave Johnson's explanation of the verse. He says that the original Greek word which has been translated into the English word "temptation" actually has a much broader meaning. More completely it means to test, to try, or to prove. But the kind of test it refers to isn't a pass or fail one. He relates it to the testing of metal by applying heat in order to draw forth from it what is pure.

The minister cites the book of Job in the Old Testament. I've tried to read Job in the past, but have always found it depressing—the suffering seems so meaningless.

He explains that before Job was tested he was a righteous, God-fearing man, a man people respected and admired. In the first chapters Job praises God in the midst of great loss. He gives all the "right spiritual responses"... "The Lord gave and the Lord hath taken away; blessed be the name of the Lord" (Job 1:21).

A glimmer of light

As I listen, I relate Job's situation to my own. During my illness, for the most part I had at least maintained a positive outward attitude. People would often comment on how strong my faith must be. Initially I felt trusting as well.

The tape continues. As Job's suffering becomes greater, his tone begins to change. He curses the day he was born (3:1), describes life as "blackness" and "terror" (3:5), wishes he had died at birth (3:11), and, like me, longs for death that does not come (3:21).

However, in the final chapters something once again causes Job's attitude to change. He affirms, "I know one thing. I know my Redeemer lives. I shall see God" (19:25). He becomes even more sure of his God and his faith than before his trials.

The pastor goes on to say, "Sometimes when God is putting you through a test, a painful thing, you don't look very good. When he's bringing forth a perfect result in you that process can be painful." Then he seems to speak directly to me. "Maybe some of you have had enough pain to hear that and go 'Baloney, you don't know what I've been through.'...I Corinthians tells us there will be a way of escape...and there hasn't been one. But sometimes the only way out of the pain you're in right now is through it, and God is not doing it to hurt you, but to call forth something that couldn't be called forth any other way, and you shall come forth as gold."

As the tape clicks off I mull over the words. They are powerful. How much I wish that I could really believe them, that eventually I will come through knowing there is a purpose in this. Haunted by my suicide attempts, I'm still unsure. At least I'm not feeling worse than before I listened to the the tape as I had expected.

Later I listen to the sermon again and am inspired. Yet, I still can't seem to move past questions that keep rolling endlessly through my mind. If God is in control and loves me, why did He allow me to come to the point that I attempted suicide? What if those attempts had worked? Would God have condemned me for trying to escape an existence that was so enormously painful I simply couldn't bear anymore and that I could see no end to?

25

November 1985 - Freedom!

I am still functioning well from an external standpoint, but my inward struggle never ends. I almost wish I could just shrug off life as a continuous chain of chance circumstances. But I'm not made that way; I analyze everything to death. I don't know how to move beyond the questioning to the point of acceptance. I know I need to do something—anything—to keep my head above water. I need to survive for Kim's sake, for the children. I've read of people being treated with hypnosis to help psychological problems. I'm unsure that it fits in with Christianity. I regard this as a last resort. As I head for the library I pray, "Dear God, I don't know if what I'm doing is right, but for over seven months I've asked for your help and guidance. If this isn't what you want then you'll have to give me an alternative."

Searching the library computer catalog through the H's and coming to "hypnosis," I find there is no shortage of books and tapes. I jot down several titles and search the shelves. At least I won't leave the library empty-handed. By the time I'm finished I have a full armload of books and tapes. My plan is to take them home to study, then talk to Jean about the idea. Maybe she'll help or at least offer a suggestion for another contact.

I'm ready to leave, but a book on an upper shelf catches my eye. *Depression* leaps from the binding. I've already read a number of books on the subject. They all seem shallow and don't identify with my situation or provide the answers I need. As I pull this one off the shelf and skim through the jacket I'm intrigued by the sub-title—*Finding Hope and Meaning in Life's Darkest Shadow*. The author is Don Baker, a Christian minister who has lived through a severe depression himself. I add it to my stack and head for the check-out counter. I wonder what the librarian is thinking as she flips open the covers and stamps in the dates one at a time.

It's four o'clock by the time I'm back home. After dinner I keep my promise to make caramel corn for the family to eat while they watch the video Kim rented. When they head off to the TV room, I clean up the kitchen and finally retreat to our bedroom and my awaiting literature. I pick up one of the books on self-hypnosis and skim a few chapters, then put it down. *Depression* has my curiosity so I delve into that.

Don Baker's description of his feelings on being admitted to a psychiatric ward hits close to home. As I read I can identify with so much of what he feels—his sense of humiliation, his fear that God has abandoned him, his belief that his life will never be normal again. Like me, he tries to pray and read the Bible, but his efforts only leave him feeling more hopeless. Even his experiences with group therapy cor-

Freedom!

relate in some respects with mine. Although he never actually attempts suicide, he comes to the point of planning how
he'd go about it, down to the location and time of day. The
fact that he is a Christian minister who had started out with
a strong faith in God makes his story especially poignant to
me. He also has a loving, supportive family.

I read on, eager to find out how Don finds his way out of
the cycle of depression and fear that continue to plague him
after he is released from the hospital. The once exuberant
pastor feels defeated, totally drained of self-confidence. His
congregation votes to let him go as pastor. He humbly accepts the offer of a friend to counsel with him on a weekly
basis.

One day Don goes to a friend's cabin to spend time
meditating and praying. In the midst of his retreat answers
finally come. His depression lifts and he is filled with so
much joy that he walks around the lake singing. Eventually
he goes on to pastor a larger church and believes that his experience with depression helps in his ministry in relating to
the problems of others.

Don's story comes like a refreshing drink to my parched
soul. This man has been where I was and where I am now
and he eventually found his way out. His life is back on an
even keel, his faith renewed.

I am drawn back to a Bible verse that was entered in the
page before Don's final chapter. "He brought me up out of
the pit of destruction, out of the miry clay; And he set my
feet upon a rock making my footsteps firm." (Psalm 40:2).
Something stirs within me—an emotion that has long eluded me is pushing its way through the shroud of fear like a
sunbeam blazing through black clouds. I get up and find a
Bible and read that verse over again. Joy is filling me with

its warmth leaving no room for fear and anxiety. I feel tears rolling down my face, but for the first time in over seven months they're cool, refreshing, cleansing, happy tears instead of tears of fear and frustration.

Freedom! The feeling is as real and dramatic as walking into a sunny blue-skied world after being held prisoner in a dank dungeon. All at once I am overflowing with love. I want to laugh and cry at the same time. Suddenly I know that God is here and has been with me all along.

Kim sees the difference immediately, the happiness mirrored in my face and my actions. He's relieved, but cautious, afraid it won't last. But days, then weeks pass and I'm staying out of the bog. My footsteps remain firm. Together we rejoice and give thanks. I have never felt the greatness of life so keenly. The whole gamut of human emotions has once again made itself available to me. I'm me again, a revitalized, rejuvenated me.

Even as I scold the children for the kinds of things mothers typically get irritated about, I'm chuckling inside and thanking God for my ability to feel and react like a normal human being—that I'm part of the world again.

When I give Don Baker's book to Jean to read she is equally impressed. Kim and I meet her for coffee and we all agree that if things should happen to take a turn for the worse I will call her, but otherwise we will resume our friendship as it was before.

On my final visit to the psychiatrist I ask Kim to come along. I've been off all the medication for a month. The psychiatrist agrees there's no reason to return. I bring the books on hypnosis back to the library unread.

26

December 1985 thru Spring 1986 - Moving ahead

When I was in the hospital I heard a lot about depression being anger turned inward. In many instances I believe there is truth in that. I still believe that the causes of my 1978 depression were a combination of built-up negative feelings and a need to continually prove myself. However, I'm convinced my recent episode was primarily drug induced. It's true that I hadn't been feeling real "up" prior to taking the Prednisone. The physical symptoms were taking their toll on myself and my family. Overall I think I was coping adequately with support from family and friends.

I haven't talked to a single doctor who doesn't agree that Prednisone use or withdrawal is capable of producing severe mental disorders. Yet, confusingly, while I was in the hospital most of the staff played down the effects of the drug.

Later one of my specialists described my experience with

total accuracy when he sympathized—"It blew your mind away, huh?"

My confusion persisted as I inquired into my medical records. I was evaluated upon admission as having "Prednisone withdrawal psychosis." Curiously, when a medication was responsible for my tortured state, my system was burdened by even more prescribed drugs. I later read that antidepressants should be used with extreme caution in patients who are in a psychotic or suicidal state, because they are capable of making the situation worse. (A psychotic state exists when a mind cannot function normally or the ability to deal with reality is impaired.) I was sent home with an entire array of pills and no one on the staff cautioned Kim or anyone else of the possible dangers for a person in my condition.

At the time I was sent home, I'd been on the antidepressant a week, not long enough to know how they were going to affect me. Most literature says it can take a month for the medication to reach full effect.

During my second hospitalization all drugs were discontinued except for a mild tranquilizer. Within the first week I was much improved, although I wasn't in a position to realize it. Then the bizarreness of what had happened and the fear it produced dominated me. At that point my "Christianity," my belief that I should have held up, added to my torment, making my suicide attempts harder to accept and put behind me. Because I was already in a weakened state and was being told repeatedly that my illness was psychological, my misery was complicated by guilt that I had failed myself and everyone else and that somehow I was responsible for my symptoms.

I have learned that no matter how much faith I have, I

Moving ahead

can't always be in control, that circumstances can still render me powerless. I don't have all the answers, I can only speak from my experiences and my own understanding. I am humbled, yet more confident in myself.

Eventually I came to be reconciled with my own suicide attempts. I read somewhere that suicide attempts are the result of a desire for attention or a desperate plea for help. Maybe in some cases this is true. But I believe often these gestures occur when a person can't comprehend that there is any other way; they are attempts to relieve agony that is too great to bear.

Depression is an illness with many different causes and it seems that the medical profession has barely tapped the surface in knowing how to adequately treat it. Depressed people need love, not judgment.

Most doctors agree that endogenous depression exists, yet they tend to become frustrated and even indignant if patients can think of nothing wrong with their external circumstances. Severe depression or psychosis can strike anyone, even those who appear emotionally strong. Drugs or biochemical imbalances within the body can create mental disorders.

Christians often find it even harder to deal with and judge themselves more harshly when depressed. They are taught they should always be cheerful, always trust God, always keep faith in adverse circumstances. If they fail, they feel their faith just isn't strong enough and it's their fault. In his book entitled "Why Christians Break Down," William A. Miller explains that often the church tells people that they are subhuman, yet expects them to act superhuman. Normal human emotions, such as anger, fear, and discouragement are expected to be suppressed. The author believes in the value of churches; he just feels that in some instances changes need to be made, and I agree.

I believe that one of the greatest gifts that God has given us is our fellow human beings. Healing so often is aided by others who have been in similar ordeals. I will always be grateful that Don Baker shared his own experience with me through his book.

I now believe that my ordeal has made me stronger emotionally and spiritually. I hit rock bottom—went beyond—and God picked me up again. I believe God was and is in my life. My faith is broader and more accepting. I see God, the world, and myself in a new light.

* * *

I have to admit that for several years I've had kind of a bah humbug attitude toward Christmas. But this Christmas of 1985 is different. It's not only a celebration of Jesus' birth, but of renewed health.

Before my severe depression, the idea that maybe I didn't want badly enough to be well gnawed at me. Now there is no question in my mind that I want to be well.

My physical symptoms remain almost in remission. Now and then slight twinges of numbness and tingling bring back thoughts of past problems, but they are minor. My gait is relatively normal, the chorea is gone and I have a fair amount of energy. I still have many unanswered questions, but I'm able to push the illness to back corners of my conciousness and to concentrate on living.

After Christmas, I half expect the usual January sluggishness, but I remain exuberant. The new year is ushered in with record amounts of snow piling up into billowing white banks. Winter has never been my favorite time of year. It always seemed easier to stay indoors than go through all the hassle of bundling up in mittens, hats, heavy jackets, and boots. This year I take advantage of every opportunity to go out and mingle with the sparkling wonderland accented by the frost-laden trees. I feel more alive than ever breathing the crisp air. Kim purchased a video camera for Christmas and he takes footage of the children tumbling into the snow banks and emerging as massive white sculptures.

One afternoon we go tobogganing with friends on a hill in the park behind our house. We swoosh down the slopes, snow billowing up in our faces, praying that the person in front will see to steer us clear of the trees at the bottom of the hill.

I've enrolled in some extension college classes that are offered in schools near our home. It is good to know that my brain still functions after twenty years of being out of an academic setting. The desire to further my education intensifies.

As the snow gradually melts I begin planning my garden. For the past several years my illness was always worse in the spring and many times I thought I would have to give up gardening. But every year I managed to work at it in bits and pieces, pacing myself. I'll be realistic this year in spite of the fact that I'm feeling quite good. As much as I enjoy the garden in the spring, by midsummer keeping it weeded and all the vegetables picked becomes endless drudgery.

By early June my life is running smoothly. I'm beginning to believe that my body has gotten the upperhand over my illness. However, it is to make one more forceful attack.

Casting all your care upon Him;
for He careth for you
1 Peter 5:7

27

July 1986 - Another battle

The couch upholstery feels coarse and bothersome, and I can't get comfortable anywhere. My body has been aching for three days with an intensity that brings back recollections of the onset of my illness five years ago. Kim is sitting next to me, his eyes fixed on the television. Suddenly my body contorts with a violent movement. Kim's eyes are drawn to me and he lets out a startled, "What the..." His voice trails off. Another violent movement sets a precedent for a continuous wave of spasms. Kim's jaw clenches and he pushes himself up from his chair without another word and storms out of the house. The back screen door slams behind him.

Jonathan rushes over and flings his arms around me. "Mom, please tell Dad to take you to the hospital!"

Jenny is in the room now too. They're both crying. I try to reassure them. "Remember, this happened before and I got better again.

"But Mom," Jonathan wails, "it wasn't this bad." He rubs a dirty hand over his tear-streaked face.

I suspect that last year's episode has magnified their fears. They now associate these symptoms with the suicide attempts. Dear God, what am I going to do? Obviously Kim isn't in a position to deal with this. Jean. I'll call Jean. Maybe she can help me figure out what to do. Please let her answer the phone.

"Hi Jean, I just need to talk to somebody. My chorea is back...the kids are crying..."

"I'll be over in just a few minutes."

Thank God for friends when I need them. After consoling the children, she sits down and we talk.

Jean is logical and calm. "Linda, in the time we spent counseling at my house, I came to some personal conclusions. Either your illness is organic or you're an extremely calculating hypochondriac and I can't believe the latter. I'll do whatever it takes to help you. I'll take time off work if necessary to accompany you to the doctor."

Kim has returned to the house and before Jean leaves she talks with him a little while. She asks Kim what he believes the problem is. His thought is still that I have some sort of fungus infestation.

Later as we lie in bed Kim distances himself from me. There may as well be a wall between us. I wish he'd put his arm around me, say something comforting. I don't know how to respond. Should I be scared? Should I be angry with Kim? I feel hurt by his apparent anger, yet I know that it's not really me that he's angry with; it's this illness. He's already been hurt too many times by it. Being callous is his way of coping now. I know that he must still have a lot of questions. Maybe he's afraid I'll go into another depression.

Another battle

I know now more than ever before that I don't want or need to be sick. I'm not bringing on this illness myself. I spent too many years questioning my sanity, fighting feelings of guilt. I won't put myself through that again. It's enough to have to cope with these symptoms. Ironically, it took the psychotic episode for me to become completely confident in my own mental soundness. Before that, I felt a certain amount of insecurity, a need to prove to the doctors and everyone around me and even to myself that I wasn't fabricating this illness for some kind of twisted personal gain. Only after every ounce of credibility had been stripped away did I reach a point where it didn't matter anymore what anyone else thought. I have stopped being afraid that I'll be rejected or abandoned. I can withstand human disapproval, secure in the love and presence of my Creator. I have come to value my belief in myself more than the opinions of others. Even if Kim has lost faith in me, I will somehow learn to live without it. But we have come this far together. I pray this episode won't drive us apart. I know I'm not to blame. I need to take a step at a time.

*Because the foolishness of God
is wiser than men;
and the weakness of God
is stronger than men.*
1 Corinthians: 1:25

28

Summer and fall 1986 - More specialists

As I hear Maxine's car pull into our driveway, I grab my purse and head out the door. She greets me as I slide into the passenger seat. "This should work out great. We'll have time to stop and pick up supplies before your appointment with Dr. Witek. Then we can stop for lunch afterward."

I am thankful that the aching is better and I'm at least back on my feet. The jerking hasn't gone away but it's much more controlled than a week ago. I'm glad that I was able to get this appointment. Dr. Witek has moved to a new clinic since I saw him a year and a half ago. It's only a few blocks from an outlet for fabric and sewing notions. Maxine doesn't mind driving me in, but I feel better knowing that we can accomplish two errands with one trip. I'm glad, too, that in spite of Jean's willingness to take off work, I don't need to rely on her.

Walking up and down the aisles at the fabric outlet quickly aggravates shortness of breath and chest pain. Any exertion lately seems to make the chorea worse. We finish in plenty of time for my appointment.

Dr. Witek hasn't changed. He is as patient and kind as I remembered. Again I feel hopeful that this doctor, who lacks the arrogance of so many of the others I've encountered, will be able to help. I feel better already, just talking with him. Nothing I say is met with indifference. I am surprised at how clear his memory is on the details of my medical history when my records are still at the other clinic and he hasn't had a chance to review them. In my experience most doctors have trouble remembering case details from one week to the next, let alone recalling medications and symptoms from over a year ago.

Dr. Witek decides to wait until completing some tests before trying any new treatments. He schedules blood work and an MRI (magnetic resonance imagery). From reading a magazine article I have learned about this new non-invasive method of viewing the inside of the body. It's been proven to be of value in detecting multiple sclerosis and other diseases, even in early stages. Dr. Witek says that if my MRI comes back normal, we can be ninety-nine percent sure I don't have multiple sclerosis. It still hasn't been completely ruled out.

Church friends offer to take me for the MRI. Kim has relaxed a little and we've talked things over. He says he will stick with me through this, but I'm relieved to have other means of transportation. I sense that it's easier for him to remain as detached as possible.

The day of the MRI is warm and sunny, not too hot for July. My friends are fun to be with and their jovial mood makes it easy for me to feel lighthearted. I still marvel that after five years they haven't given up on me.

The MRI involves being placed on a cradle and inserted into a narrow cylindrical hole within a huge magnet. The attending nurse puts cotton in my ears and a black cloth over my face to shut out as much stimulation as possible and calm my movement. For an hour I am lulled into a semi-sleep by a soft knocking sound. When a voice finally announces that the test is almost done, I reach up and pull away the cloth and am surprised to see myself reflected in a mirror just inches from my face. There are mirrors on either side, too. Though not usually claustrophobic, I'm more than ready to get out by the time they are finished.

Dr. Witek is always prompt in calling me personally to inform me of test results. He reports that the MRI was unrevealing. The blood tests are normal except for a slightly elevated strep titer, which could indicate a recent infection. Dr. Schrock once commented that my chorea may be strep related. I was aware of swollen glands a few days ago, along with a slight fever. Off and on over the years I have noted that a low grade fever accompanies the more acute flare-ups of my problems.

Dr. Witek isn't ready to give up. He arranges for another EEG before referring me to two other specialists, a rheumatologist and another neurologist. The former asks if I've ever been tested for Lyme disease. When I tell him I have, he admits he's baffled. The latter decides my movement isn't chorea, but tremors (which she pronounces as "treemers"). She has no answers for me either and says that any other tests she can think of would be dangerous and probably a disservice to me.

Because Dr. Witek thinks I should be in contact with an internist, I've put myself under the care of Dr. Robert

LYME DISEASE: My Search for a Diagnosis

Needham. He has been helpful and encouraging. He's explained that although we like to put things into neat little
categories and have names for them, sometimes that isn't
possible. Although all my symptoms indicate the strong
possibility of a collagen vascular disease, they don't fit the
pattern of any particular known one.

* * *

The children seem to have adjusted well to my condition—even the movement. In mid-summer a former
neighbor and close friend returns from Chicago to Minnesota for a visit and I bring Jason, Jenny, and Jonathan
along to see her. My chorea is active, but manageable
enough to drive. Jason confides that it scared him a little to
ride with me until he realized that I did fine and knew when
I shouldn't drive. Jenny says that she decribes my problems
to her friends before they come to our house so they won't be
alarmed when they see my chorea for the first time. Last
year my children seemed to feel awkward and embarrassed;
now they are able to deal with it honestly and openly. I'm
proud of them. They can even kid about it. On the way to my
friend's house, Jenny wonders aloud how my friend will
react when she sees me. "I know," Jonathan says. "Why
don't we all do what Mom's doing, then she won't feel so
funny." All three attempt to imitate my gyrations, laughing
themselves silly in the process. They make me feel good.

On the serious side, I learn from Jennifer's teachers that
she has been asking questions about collagen diseases and
other illnesses she's heard mentioned and trying to find
related articles in the library. One day, out of the clear blue,
she asks if I have cancer. When I assure her that I don't she

- 174 -

breathes a heavy sigh of relief. She, too, is trying hard to understand what is happening.

* * *

Later in the fall Jean offers to take me with her to the biomedical library at the University of Minnesota. While she works on a research paper, I spend several hours looking up information on collagen diseases. Many of the case histories are written in foreign languages. One that is in English presents a victim who has the same kind of pinpoint hemorrhages inside the bladder that my medical records indicate I've had. I note that many of the collagen diseases are fatal. The treatments suggested are invariably steroids. Since my bad experience with Prednisone, I don't see them as being an option in my case.

On the way home Jean asks what kind of conclusions I've drawn. I respond that from everything I've read all my symptoms do fit into the collagen vascular disease category except that most of the people I read about weren't functioning nearly as well as I am. I'm not sick enough. The pieces still don't quite fit.

Further elaborate testing on my bladder indicates significant dysfunction of the nerves and muscles. I am told by the urologist that the problem is most likely stemming from the brain or spinal cord. This information further convinces me that there is a connection between the bladder symptoms and the other neurological problems.

At times I think that Dr. Witek is more determined than I am to solve this puzzle. He racks his brain trying to think of anything he might have missed. He would like me to go to the Mayo Clinic, but he's prescribed an anti-seizure drug once again and it's controlling the movement fairly well. Right now I've had my fill of doctors and tests and still no answers. It isn't until later in the fall, when I develop an allergy to the medication, that I agree to go.

29

December 1986 - A week at the Mayo

My appointment at the Mayo is arranged for the first week in December. Before going I request and receive copies of my medical records from several of the doctors I've consulted over the years. After reading through them I am dismayed and angered by inconsistencies and inaccuracies I discover in many of them dating back to the first year of my illness. Statements about my earlier "psychiatric" problems are grossly exaggerated and often the information doesn't correlate with what the physicians had related to Kim and me.

In 1981 one doctor had recorded that I have a "strong history of severe somatic complaints with no physiological basis." He also wrote that for years I'd had "annual episodes of crying jags, tremors, and irritability, etc." Neither statement has any supporting data for his conclusions. Kim and I have been together for over twenty years and he is upset, too, by these statements. This doesn't sound like the Linda he knows. My one spell involving crying jags had not been accompanied by other physical symptoms.

I write this doctor a seven page letter explaining my objections to these and many other ungrounded assertions. Before I even mail it I call to confirm how angry I am. At first he becomes defensive and I find myself practically yelling at him. Meek, passive, always follow-the-doctors-orders little me!

Realizing that much of the false information has been passed on to other doctors infuriates me even more. I wonder how differently my medical investigation might have progressed if I had sought out my records earlier. How much money could have been saved? Pain avoided?

We have paid out enormous sums of money for medical expenses over the years. As a result of recorded inaccuracies others may have favored a psychosomatic explanation. I, too, had almost become convinced I was crazy.

After nearly an hour's conversation, the doctor doesn't come up with any explanation for his blunders, but he finally admits that he owes me a "gigantic apology" and offers to add my letter to my records with a signed statement from him saying that it is a better account of my medical history than his own entries.

Another doctor stated that I'd been under psychiatric care "for years" prior to consulting him, but the "patient did not admit this initially." I never admitted this to him because it just isn't true! When questioned he, too, is unable to justify his statment.

Other early records proclaim that my MMPI showed a "severely hysterical personality." No one bothered to record that further testing and interviews showed normal findings and a stable personality. When I try to obtain copies of the original questionnaire and graphing of the abnormalities, I learn that they have mysteriously vanished from my file at the originating clinic.

A final insult comes when I learn the psychiatrist I visited six times following my last hospitalization entered no information in his charts other than the date. There is nothing on record to indicate that I had ever recovered from the Prednisone depression.

I call several psychologists who all confirm that they believe the Rorschach test would be more valuable than the MMPI in a case like mine. I also talk to Grant Dahlstrom, who heads the Department of Psychology at the University of North Carolina and has co-authored two handbooks on the use of the MMPI. He states that it is expecting too much of the test to be able to determine if physical symptoms are psychological and that it should be used with extreme caution in these situations, and only in conjunction with other tests.

Many records also list several organic possibilities that I was never told about. Some extremely rare and sometimes fatal neurological diseases, including Huntington's, are mentioned. One CAT scan of the brain showed "increased atrophy, which can sometimes be seen in degenerative diseases." At the time I was told it was normal.

* * *

I have most of the records in hand when we head for the Mayo. Kim isn't thrilled about going, but he has agreed to drive me there and stay the first day. Then Nancy, a friend who lives in Rochester, will pick me up and bring me to stay at her house between tests and appointments.

My first appointment is at 7 a.m. and we leave by 5 o'clock. It's snowing and the roads are glazed with ice. I pray that the weather won't pose any problems. Dr. Witek has arranged for me to meet Dr. Drake Duane, a neurologist who specializes in movement disorders. I've only gotten in because of a cancellation. If we miss this appointment there'll be no more openings for several months. I'm trying to think positively, but I'm afraid this will turn out to be another wild goose chase. In spite of the Mayo reputation for having the best facilities available and the fact that many people come from all over the world to be treated here, I've heard stories of unpleasant experiences. Yet family members have urged me to come for so long. If nothing else, this may put their minds at ease. They'll know every avenue has been explored.

In my head I begin counting doctors. "Kim do you realize that, as nearly as I can figure, I've seen twenty-seven doctors in the past five and a half years and we're no closer to an answer than we started."

"Well, I'm worried that you're getting your hopes up again and will be depressed if this trip fails to turn up anything," Kim says.

"It's something I just have to get through. I'll be disappointed, but I'll get over it."

As we near Rochester, the sun is shining over the horizon and the ice on the main roads has melted from the traffic.

The Mayo Clinic rises majestically above the other buildings in the center of the city. Three dimensional figures of a man, woman, and child project from the granite front. We locate a parking ramp, then make our way to the main

A week at the Mayo

lobby to check in and fill out insurance forms and medical questionnaires. The neurology clinic is on the eighth floor. Rows of seats fill a huge waiting area, reminding me more of a bus depot than a medical clinic. We speak to a receptionist and sit down to wait our turn. After a restless hour I hear my name called over the speaker. When Kim gets up to follow me, a nurse halts him by the entrance to the office area. "Dr. Duane would like to talk to her alone first."

She leads me down a hallway and gestures that I be seated on a leather couch in an examing room. A large desk to my right is piled with stacks of papers and unopened mail. My nervousness is making the chorea more pronounced, which is fine with me. I'd rather have the doctor see my symptoms at their worst than try to describe them. My head moves side to side and my body jerks harshly and repetitively to the right. I pull one magazine after another off a rack next to the couch, flipping through the pages without seeing much of anything.

A tap on the door brings my heart to my throat. I've gathered that this man I'm about to meet is probably as knowledgeable as anyone in the world about the speciality of movement disorders. Tall and rugged looking, Dr. Duane enters and walks by me, barely pausing to shake my hand. I'm not even sure he looked at me. He seats himself in a swivel chair and becomes engrossed in a sheaf of papers he picks up from his desk. He pulls out a letter that I'm close enough to recognize as Dr. Witek's. It doesn't appear that he's familiarized himself with my case before now. As he continues paging through my records, he is interrupted by several phone calls. I'm beginning to think that he's forgotten I'm here.

Finally he turns toward me. After a few minutes of conversation his initial brusque manner dissolves and I begin to like him.

"I see that it's been suggested that your symptoms might be psychosomatic. How do you feel about that?"

"I can't deny that I've had some emotional problems, but I can't believe that I'm neurotic enough to come up with all these symptoms," I reply.

"Well, you're right. This is definitely an organic problem, not a psychological one."

I wasn't expecting him to express such strong confidence in that fact so early in the interview. He seems as certain as Dr. Witek was after our first encounter three years ago. At least I won't have to contend with another doctor's insistence that I need psychiatric care. He jots notes as he goes and makes some phone calls giving people instructions on tests he is scheduling. He seems sure of himself, yet not condescending or arrogant, and genuinely interested in my comments and questions.

"I'd like to have your movement videotaped so we can study it more closely, but we'll need to have consent forms signed. I'm sure that we'll be able to help you and hopefully come up with a diagnosis before you leave."

Twenty minutes later I am handed a folder containing my test schedule for the next five days. I'm impressed with the speed and efficiency with which they've been arranged.

When Nancy picks me up at five o'clock Kim heads back home. He will return after the tests are completed. Nancy's lively personality is a morale booster. She and her husband make me feel welcome in their home. She cheerfully drives me back to the clinic each day.

Many of the tests are repeats of ones that have been done already, but some are more elaborate. One EEG consists of electrodes being fastened to my head first, then attached to the entire right side of my body. Two technicians and a doctor work on me for nearly three hours before the test is completed. While they are all busy figuring out where to fasten the electrodes, I happen to spot my chart sitting on a nearby table. I can't resist picking it up and reading what Dr. Duane has written, and no one seems to mind. His impression is that I have some sort of central nervous system disease, but is not sure of its exact nature. He also comments that "this woman is bright, intuitive, and analytical." What a pleasant offset to some of the remarks made about me in some past records.

Making the video entails a more elaborate setup than I'd anticipated. I walk into what makes me think of a TV studio. Clothed in undergarments, I make my film debut sitting, standing, and lying down. I'm asked to read aloud a selection of prose to reveal any speech problems.

Several EMGs (electromyograms) send painful jolts of electricity through almost every part of my body. These tests measure the speed of nerve conduction and the electrical activity of muscle fibers. I've had similar tests in the past on my arms and legs. But I don't ever recall the shocks being so intense and painful. It's one series I hope not to have repeated.

On the fifth and final day, I am in the physical medicine department. Dr. Duane has suggested that a small electrical device, which produces electrical vibrations, might be worth trying in an attempt to control the jerking, which he has now redefined, as dystonic dyskinesia.

The female technician is patiently explaining how the device, called a TENS unit, works. "The electrical vibrations somehow block the signals the brain is sending to certain areas of your body. We place the electrodes near the problem areas, but we're not sure where to put them. We have to just use the trial and error method."

I'm not in any mood for this. I'm tired of being poked and prodded and wired to machines and I can't believe that this little gadget will have any effect on my movement.

The technician tapes two electrodes to my right side and two others just below the back of my neck. "You can adjust the setting yourself to whatever is comfortable," she says. As I experiment with the dial, a series of racing shocks tingle the surface of my skin.

"Just leave it on for awhile. The effects tend to be accumulative, which means they may be more effective after it's turned off again," she explains. When the TENS is shut off after about twenty minutes, my movement is barely noticeable. To the amazement of both of us this thing is working!

Kim returns in time to sit in on the final verdict. Dr. Duane is pulling on a coat as he walks in the door. He sits on the edge of his chair and talks rapidly.

"After reviewing all the tests I am convinced your movement disorder is being caused by a Parkinsonian type disorder. You don't have Parkinson's disease itself; however, your problem is being produced by a chemical imbalance within the brain similar to that which occurs with Parkinson's. We have no way of knowing whether this will get worse or not. I'll send copies of my evaluations to you and to Dr. Witek."

With that, he is getting up to leave again. We haven't had a chance to ask questions, but I don't want to make Dr. Duane late for whatever he's hurrying off to.

We leave the Mayo with mixed emotions. On the way out

we stop at the pharmacy and purchase the $600 TENS unit which Dr. Duane has prescribed. I am grateful that this device, combined with the medication I'm already taking, is helping tremendously. Dr. Duane also says he will send a list of medications for future trial should I need them. My disappointment in not receiving a name for my illness gradually eases into acceptance of the fact that I'll probably never have one. At this point I try to find consolation by telling myself it doesn't really matter. Having a diagnosis most likely won't change anything. From everything I've read, most neurological diseases have no cure anyway.

*My grace is sufficient
for thee: for my strength
is made perfect in weakness*
2 Corinthians 12:9

30

Spring and summer 1987 - Acceptance

It's been six years since the onset of my illness. My condition has worsened since my December 1986 trip to the Mayo Clinic. Earlier in the spring Dr. Witek prescribed a wheelchair because of the extreme difficulty I have walking distances. Sometimes even half a block will do me in. I become out of breath with the slightest exertion and my chest hurts all the time. Rather than purchasing a wheelchair, I borrow one. I dislike the contraption more than I thought I would. It's an ugly combination of green vinyl and metal and it's awkward and clumsy. Yet, if it means I can get out instead of staying home, I'll use it.

In May Dr. Witek arranges for a second consultation at the Mayo and Dr. Duane notes that there has been progression since he last saw me. My right foot pulls inward—so tightly most of the time that it hurts and it's almost impossible to straighten. My movement is going beyond the capacity of the TENS unit to control. More muscles are involved, pulling against each other painfully, sometimes causing my back to arch. They seem to want to twist my body in every direction at once. Occasionally there is noticeable twitching in my right arm and that worries me. Until now I've had full control in both arms. Dr. Duane brings up the possibility of experimental spinal cord surgery, but only after more medication trials. I am also confronted by a therapist in the physical medicine department, who begins discussing various aids for the handicapped—canes, walkers, safety devices for the bathroom. I find myself wanting to put my hands over my ears and shut out what she is saying.

Dr. Duane says that my breathlessness is probably caused by involvement of the diaphragm. The nerves and muscles to my bladder are functioning so poorly that I am using a catheter. My body appears to be weakening against the monster that continues to attack it.

* * *

The end of May brings Jerimiah's high school graduation and we throw a party to celebrate. Friends and relatives come over to wash windows and help with other tasks that are too exhausting for me. They also prepare a good share of the food. With so many helping hands the party goes smoothly. Over a hundred people come to share the occasion and afterward many send notes saying how much they enjoyed the event.

A few days later Jason, our adventurer, boards a plane for Indonesia as a foreign exchange student. The emotional stress of the combined events puts me in bed for three days.

Acceptance

My balance is so far off that I can't get up without supporting myself against a wall. I have a good long cry, partly out of sentiment that two of my children are practically adults, partly from apprehension. What kind of physical shape will I be in by the time the others are ready to graduate? I'm never sure when things are going to get bizarre. Although I realize that life is uncertain for everyone. I am reminded of that uncertainty constantly. When I do start feeling self-pity, I remind myself that life isn't a piece of cake for anyone. Those who have their health often struggle with a multitude of other stresses.

I am especially confident of and most thankful for my sanity. The verse that has come to mind so often during the past years is real to me. *For God hath not given us the spirit of fear; but of power, and of love, and of a sound mind.* (2 Timothy 1:7). The dictionary defines power as the ability to act. In spite of my weaknesses I believe that I have the ability to act—to make decisions concerning my medical care as well as other areas in my life. I will stand by my beliefs. I know my body and mind better than any other human being. I feel emotionally well, surrounded by love, and am unafraid to face the future, whatever it may hold.

I don't know how to account for others who are struggling with chronic emotional problems. I can only offer my compassion and prayers and the hope that God will eventually restore them and give the peace that I have been blessed with.

*But they that wait upon the Lord
shall renew their strength; they
shall mount up with wings as eagles;
they shall run, and not be weary;
and they shall walk, and not faint*
Isaiah 40:31

31

Autumn 1987 - A diagnosis!

I managed to work at the shop through the summer, yet I was often rendered helpless when the heat was more extreme. It was the first summer I made no attempt to plant a garden.

I've started thinking more about the future. I've continued taking some extension classes, but am unsure what kinds of goals to set. I don't have any idea what I'll be capable of doing. The way things look I'd better choose work that I could carry on from a wheelchair, if necessary. My right arm is becoming increasingly twitchy, my right foot is crooked at an angle most of the time and more and more the left is imitating it.

By early October, on the third anniversary of our opening, I resign myself to moving my business back home. It's a wrenching decision. For the most part the venture has been a good experience. I was hoping to wait at least until after Christmas, but I'm unable to keep up with the work load and find myself frustrated as a result. I seldom make it through a whole day. Kim and Jerimiah often need to pick me up or Maxine must interrupt her work to drive me home.

Our TV room becomes my sewing room. At home I can sew for a couple of hours, then lie down and rest. But I miss the conversation, so I keep the TV on in the morning for company. Once in awhile an interesting topic arises.

On a local talk show, they are discussing the Epstein-Barr virus, a chronic fatigue syndrome caused by the same organism that produces mononucleosis. My ears perk up when I hear medical subjects being discussed.

Before the commercial break, they mention that an infectious disease specialist will appear. The thought crosses my mind that maybe it could be the one who cared for me in 1985. I go to the refrigerator for a glass of milk and return to see Dr. Schrock's familiar face on the screen. Guests on the show are talking about typical symptoms of Epstein-Barr—fatigue, aching, headache. Dr. Schrock mentions something about neurological symptoms, but I missed part of it. I know the Epstein-Barr virus is something I've never been tested for. Even though my symptoms don't all fit it may be worth checking out.

The program is over and I'm dialing Dr. Schrock's number for an appointment. Maybe this is silly. I have an appointment with Dr. Witek next week. If he thinks this is pointless I can always cancel it.

However, Dr. Witek encourages me to follow through with this, saying that Dr. Schrock would have more knowledge in the area of Epstein-Barr virus infections. It's typical of him not to brush anything off. I'm not sure I would have continued to search for an answer without his continued encouragement and support.

A diagnosis!

Dr. Schrock agrees to test me for antibodies to the Epstein-Barr virus, and says he also wants to check for Lyme disease.

"I was already tested for Lyme disease before," I protest. Only then do I learn the Lyme test was never completed. Dr. Schrock tells me that, although the blood was drawn and sent to the state lab in 1985, he had received a letter back stating that the test wasn't available in Minnesota at the time.

"Well, I'm sure that either Dr. Witek or the Mayo has checked it again. They've been so thorough. I know it's been mentioned and every other test has been repeated."

"I'd like to do it anyway, so I can see for myself," Dr. Schrock insists.

I chide myself as I leave the office. Why do I keep putting myself through this? I know that nothing will come of these tests. They're a waste of time and money. I'm irritated with myself for coming, and at Dr. Schrock for insisting on additional blood work.

I phone Dr. Witek when I return home. He's surprised that the Lyme test was never actually done. He has never ordered a repeat himself because there was no evidence in the records he received that it hadn't been completed the first time. Looking back over my Mayo records, I see no indication that it was checked there, either. I still don't think too much of it. I'm not really sure what Lyme disease is. In all the reading I've done in the past six years I don't recall any literature on it. But as I mull it over, something clicks in my mind. My sister-in-law, Jan, did pass along a newspaper clipping last spring about a woman with an unusual illness. Maybe it was this one. I can't recall if I saved the article or not, but I begin searching through stacks of papers on my closet shelves. I find it tucked underneath other articles about nutrition, depression and an assortment of other illnesses. I remember that on first reading it, I noticed quite a few similarities between the woman's condition and my own. But my illness had seemed similar to so many others over the years, and because I was so certain I'd been tested for Lyme disease, I dismissed it entirely. I reread the article now with a little more interest. The woman lives in Plymouth, a town about twenty miles from us. Her illness had started like mine—fatigue, chills, aching joints, chest pain. Her ensuing neurological symptoms led doctors to believe she had multiple sclerosis, but nothing turned up on tests. Her husband, a hospital chemist, learned of Lyme disease and decided she should be tested. The article indicated that following treatment her condition improved significantly.

According to the article, Lyme disease is caused by deer ticks, which thrive wherever there are deer.

Her husband's name is mentioned in the article, so I have no trouble locating the number in the telephone book. I hope my call won't be an intrusion.

A chipper voice answers the phone. I've reached Sondra, the woman in the article. She's happy to talk to me when I explain why I'm calling and is very interested in my story.

"My husband was the one who pursued testing and arranged to send blood samples to three different labs. Each one came out different. One came back negative, one borderline, and one highly positive for Lyme disease, " she patiently explains. "The tests aren't always accurate, so don't let them base their decision on one blood test alone."

Maybe, just maybe, there is a chance my blood test will turn something up. But what if it doesn't? Will Dr. Schrock

A diagnosis!

think that it might be worth repeating the test or trying the treatment for Lyme disease regardless?

Now I'm getting more anxious to hear from Dr. Schrock, but a week has gone by and still no word. He said I should call in two weeks if I didn't hear from him.

It's not quite two weeks yet, but I can't stand the suspense any longer and I phone Dr. Schrock's office. The nurse takes a message for him to return my call, but I wait all day beside a silent phone. I call again the next morning. Once more the nurse answers.

"Please, I just want to know the results of my blood test."

Good, she's going to check. She's back on the line. "Well...I think I'd better have Dr. Schrock call and explain this to you."

I'm impatient. "But you would tell me if they were negative, wouldn't you?"

"I'm just not sure how to interpret what they have written here. Your titer was 1:64. And it says here if a current infection is suspected to have it retested in about three weeks."

When I hang up my head is whirling. Apparently the test wasn't negative...but I don't know what a 1:64 titer means. Maybe it's low but not negative. Sondra's words ring in my ears. "The tests aren't always accurate. Don't rely on one blood test."

I don't want to be a nuisance, but I call Sondra again. This time she puts her husband on the phone.

He seems convinced from everything I've told him that there's a good enough chance that I do have Lyme disease that I should be treated for it. He explains that a titer measures the level of antibodies in the blood and that although my titer was low it proved that I'd been exposed to the Lyme bacteria at some time. Titers tend to drop over a period of years even though the patient may still have live spirochetes in his system creating internal havoc.

I receive articles about Lyme disease in the mail from Sondra and from my mother-in-law. Every one of my symptoms fits. We have deer and ticks in our area and so far nothing else conclusive has turned up. This has to be my answer. It has to! I call Dr. Russell Johnson, a professor of microbiology at the University of Minnesota, who authored one of the articles. He has been researching Lyme disease for a number of years and agrees that other people with low and even negative titers have been proven to have Lyme disease spirochetes in their bodies.

From everything I read, Lyme disease is presumed to be very treatable with antibiotics in the early stages, but if left untreated too long symptoms may be irreversible. After more than six years will mine be too late to treat? Up until the past year I've had partial remissions. That might be a good sign. Even if my symptoms can't be reversed I know I want to be treated, if only to prevent further progression. If that's all I can hope for, it's still a lot!

When Kim comes home I choke on my words before I finally get them out. "Oh Kim! I know this is what it is. I just know it! But what if Dr. Schrock doesn't agree?"

Finally on Friday, Dr. Schrock returns my call. He says he's not convinced my Lyme titer is high enough to warrant treatment, but readily agrees to try it considering my symptoms and our location near the park reserve. He warns me that it's expensive and that he'll have to check to make sure our insurance will cover a portion of it. He'll set up a date to start an IV treatment next week.

In the meantime Kim leaves for deer hunting. When

A diagnosis!

friends of Kim's family drive me to Dr. Schrock's office my symptoms are at their worst. Dr. Schrock has suddenly become more enthusiastic about the treatment than he had been over the phone. He says that just the evening prior to my appointment he attended a Lyme disease seminar and learned that the chemist was right about the blood titer—a low result is irrelevant in the face of so many typical symptoms. He says that the disease is known to affect the bladder as mine has been, and that chorea is seen with Lyme disease as well.

With an intern and a nurse observing, Dr. Schrock attempts to insert a long plastic tube in my lower left arm. After a struggle with tricky veins and a switch to my right arm the catheter is inserted through my arm and shoulder and into my chest. An x-ray is taken to insure proper positioning. A nurse demonstrates how to drain medication into my vein. Twice a day for two weeks I am to hook myself up to a bag containing high doses of an antibiotic called Rocephin (ceftriaxone). I've learned from my reading that it's more effective in wiping out Lyme disease spirochetes than other antibiotics.

I'm thankful, so thankful that Dr. Schrock has agreed to try this. I have no idea what to expect. I don't anticipate any change for at least several weeks. Sondra said her condition hadn't improved until she was off the medication for several months. A sister of a friend, is being treated for the second time and still isn't feeling better.

Dr. Witek calls and cautions me not to get my hopes too high. I really only dare hope that the Rocephin will keep my symptoms from worsening and promote even slight improvement in the way I'm feeling.

* * *

LYME DISEASE: My Search for a Diagnosis

It's the middle of the third day of treatment. Jennifer has appointed herself my nurse, helping me hook up the bags of medication and regulate the pace of the flow. She's ecstatic about the possibility of my being diagnosed. Only ten grams of Rocephin, two grams at a time, have dripped their way slowly into my bloodstream. It's too soon to be feeling as good as I am. But since this morning I haven't had a trace of the involuntary muscle movements and I haven't used the TENS unit at all. I keep waiting for them to resume, but they don't. My right foot is relaxed and straight; I'm not fighting to keep it from pulling inward. I tap it over and over. For almost a year there has never been a time I could coordinate my foot to accomplish this task. My left foot, which has lately been recalcitrant is behaving,too. I'm scared. So scared. I don't want to say anything to anyone else. People keep calling to see how I'm doing. "Better," I say. I downplay this. I can't believe it's really working this fast and I don't want to get everyone's hopes up.

The next morning I wake to a calm, relaxed body—no twitching, no jerking, no pain! I'm excited! It's a Sunday late in November. I go outside. The air is frigid, the sky overcast, but I feel alive and energetic. I walk easily with a coordinated gait. How unfamiliar not to struggle with every step. Even the cold air being drawn into my lungs doesn't bring chest pain and shortness of breath.

A mile later I'm home again, flying back into the house, hugging Kim, dancing around the room. "Kim, look at me! Can you believe it? I've just walked a mile and I still have energy to spare!"

I sit down and make my foot move freely in every direction. This is all so much more than I had hoped for or even dreamed possible. Jenny is as giddy with excitement as I

A diagnosis!

am and she and Jonathan spend the next day at school announcing the good news to all their friends and teachers.

* * *

On November 25th, 1987, one day before Thanksgiving, I return to have my catheter removed.

Dr. Schrock is beaming when he sees how well I am.

"Does this mean that I have a real diagnosis?"

"Yes. I think it's safe to assume that Lyme disease was causing your problems."

I am still not sure this isn't all a dream. Oh God, thank you! I can't believe it! After six and a half years I have *both* a diagnosis and a treatment that works! If I pinch myself will this turn out to be a fantasy? I am pinching myself mentally and it isn't a dream. It's real!

I think back on the past years. Some doctors told me that I was better off with no diagnosis, because it would probably only mean that the illness was advancing and there was little that could be done to stop it anyway. It's ironic. All the tests, all the high tech equipment, and it took a simple blood test to pinpoint the cause.

Now that I have the answer, every piece of the puzzle fits. Lyme disease is capable of causing an incredibly vast array of symptoms.

Lyme disease spirochetes can work their way into many areas of the body, producing inflammation and pain. The heart, lungs, bladder, brain, joints and nerves are often affected. Symptoms may come and go, one flaring unexpectedly, another going inexplicably dormant. As the body produces antibodies and reactive cells to fight the spirochetes, symptoms can show up in many places and many times at unpredictable intervals.

My uncontrollable movement, difficulty walking, poor bladder control, halting speech and loss of balance must all have been a result of spirochete invasion in the areas of the brain that regulated those funtions.

My joint and muscle pain, along with some inflammation in the rib joints, wrists and occasionally in my hands, also fit the illness. Pleurisy, low grade fever, and heart palpitations are other common symptoms. The numbness and tingling, the weakness and fatigue probably indicated the nerves themselves were being attacked by the spirochetes.

Although Lyme disease can also affect the areas of the brain that control mood and memory, resulting in depression, psychotic derangement, and dementia, I believe that my psychotic episode and ensuing depression were a direct result of the medication, not the Lyme disease. The incident occurred after I was given the Prednisone and it was the only time during the six-year ordeal that I experienced that type of problem.

For so many years I woke up every morning conscious of the fact that I was ill. Now when I wake up I am aware that I am well!

* * *

On Thanksgiving Eve I am sitting in a pew in the front row of our little church, emotion welling up within me. I'm surrounded by people who have prayed for me faithfully during my years of struggle with Lyme disease. When I was ready to give up they wouldn't let me. They encouraged me, consoled me, and became angry for me. They believed in me

A diagnosis!

when I didn't believe in myself. Because of them, I've learned to be more open to the needs of others. At times they literally became my strength and my faith and now, because of the way God worked through them, I believe I have love, faith, and strength to give back.

This evening I have asked for a few minutes to get up and share my thankfulness for my renewed health and to thank everyone for their prayers. It's not common for me to carry a Bible to church. I've brought Kim's Bible to hold, just for security. As a visiting minister reads Psalm 103, I follow along. The third verse is highlighted with a pencil. Kim must have marked it years earlier during Sunday school class. *Bless the Lord...Who forgives all your iniquity, who heals all your diseases.*

For that verse to stand out now couldn't be more appropriate. It reminds me that, even though it was the doctors who eventually diagnosed and treated me, God is the instigator of all healing. In six years I went from faith to uncertainty—almost lost my faith completely. But God came through.

I sense that this is an end and a beginning. There are so many things I thought I wouldn't be able to do. I can say thank you a thousand times and it will never be enough! I have grown through all the doubt and fear and the disillusionment. I have been blessed! I would never have believed that there would come a time when I could look back and say it was worth the suffering. Yet, I know now that it has been. I know that my healing and its timing have been perfect!

But he knows the way that I take; when he has tried me, I shall come forth as gold! (Job 23:10).

EPILOGUE

I returned to Dr. Witek a few months following my treatment and he agreed with Dr. Schrock's diagnosis of Lyme disease. It has now been nearly three years since I was treated with antibiotics. My energy level is equal to what it was before my illness began in 1981. Since my treatment I have had no chorea, no speech problems, no heart palpitations, and no aching. My gait and balance have remained normal. My bladder symptoms and head discomfort left more slowly, but are now so minor they are hardly worth mentioning.

During the past three years I have had the opportunity to speak to various organizations and at medical conferences around the United States. The feedback I receive from lay people and from those in the medical profession continually reinforces my belief that there is a great need for better understanding of the emotional impact of dealing with difficult-to-diagnose illness. In response to that need I have written a second book titled *When You're Sick and Don't Know Why*(DCI Publishing 1991), which is a self-help book for those coping with undiagnosed illness.

Looking back on my own six years of undiagnosed illness, I can honestly say that I don't regret anything that happened. Although it was immensely frightening and painful at times, I gained insights never anticipated, anchored my spiritual beliefs beyond expectation and discovered wonderful qualities in human relationships. Had my disease been diagnosed soon after I contracted it, I would have missed these opportunities and no doubt never would have written this book.

In the following sections I have organized what I have learned into five main topics and, in each, have summarized my personal thoughts.

LYME DISEASE: My Search for a Diagnosis

FACTS ABOUT LYME DISEASE
"If it weren't for AIDS (acquired immune deficiency syndrome), Lyme disease would be the number one new disease facing us today."
— *Russell C. Johnson, Ph.D.*

Dr. Russell C. Johnson is a professor of microbiology in the School of Medicine at the University of Minnesota in Minneapolis. He is well-known for his research in Lyme disease and has confirmed the following facts:

Lyme disease is a multisystem bacterial illness transmitted most often by the painless bite of a tiny tick commonly referred to as a deer tick. Other ticks known to carry the disease are the California black-legged tick and the lone star tick.

Lyme disease is becoming increasingly prevalent and is currently the most common tick-borne illness in the United States. Although first described in 1909 in European medical journals, the first outbreak in the United States was noted in 1975 by two mothers from Lyme, Connecticut. Six years later Dr. Willy Burgdorfer, a scientist at the Rocky Mountain Labs, identified the pathogen as a corkscrew-shaped bacterium which is now known as *Borrelia burgdorferi.*

Endemic areas include the northeastern states of Connecticut, New York, New Jersey, Massachusetts, and Rhode Island; the north central states of Minnesota and Wisconsin; the western states of California, Oregon, Utah, and Nevada; and the central northeastern portion of Texas.

Deer, rodents and other animals serve as hosts to the tick during various stages of its life cycle. Infected ticks are car-

Epilogue

ried to new areas by birds and mammals and have been found in woods, beaches and front yards.

The deer tick may transmit the infection during the adult stage. However, it more commonly causes problems while still in the nymph stage when it is no bigger than a pin head. The nymphs are active in the spring and summer when people wear little protective clothing and are likely to be camping or hiking in the woods. The tick attaches itself to its victim where it remains until engorged, then falls off. A deer tick bite does not always result in Lyme disease.

Symptoms may vary greatly from person to person. Some, but not all, bites result in a ring-shaped rash at the occurring site. These are the cases most likely to be diagnosed early. A flu-like illness is common at the onset—chills, fever, aching, stiff neck, weakness and fatigue. Other symptoms which can follow immediately or occur months or years later may include weight loss, arthritis, heart palpitations, depression, chest pain, numbness, facial palsy, speech impairment, eye problems, stomach problems, chorea, balance and coordination problems, bladder difficulties, paralysis, and dementia.

Lyme disease is treatable with antibiotics. However, because it imitates and is often mistaken for other maladies such as multiple sclerosis, rheumatoid arthritis, lupus, and various psychiatric disorders, many people who could be helped by treatment aren't receiving it. The disease affects both sexes and all age groups. It may also be passed on to the fetus in a pregnant woman.

Prompt diagnosis and treatment are important because treatment is most effective in early stages. Early Lyme disease may be treated with oral antibiotics. However, high doses of intravenous antibiotics are often necessary to com-

LYME DISEASE: My Search for a Diagnosis

pletely knock out the bacteria in people who have chronic signs of the disease. Even then, not all victims respond to treatment.

Diagnosing Lyme disease can be difficult. Serologic testing methods are still fairly new and not highly accurate. Results may vary from laboratory to laboratory and patient antibody response varies greatly. A common mistake is interpreting low blood titers as negative for Lyme disease when, in fact, people with low blood titers can have active infections producing severe symptoms. Dr. Johnson considers IFA titers of 1:64 or higher as evidence of Lyme disease in patients who are experiencing symptoms typical of the disease. (The test measures how aggressively the person's body is producing antibodies to the spirochetes.) He reports that approximately 50 percent of the victims have negative titers during early stages of the disease. Therefore, he believes that the diagnosis of Lyme disease should be based primarily on clinical manifestations, using serology to confirm the conclusion.

Lyme antibodies may be present in synovial and cerebral spinal fluid of patients who have arthritic and neurologic manifestations. Therefore in some cases spinal taps may be beneficial in diagnosing the illness. Some, who have had negative blood titers, have had positive spinal fluid titers.

The MIDWESTERN LYME ASSOCIATION provides information on support groups, physicians and educational resources : Midwestern Lyme Association, 3835 S. 37th, Lincoln, Nebraska 68506. (402) 475-4011.

The LYME BORRELIOSIS FOUNDATION sponsors public education, medical conferences, publications and research: Lyme Borreliosis Foundation, Inc. P.O. Box 462, Tolland, CT O6084. (203) 871-2900.

Epilogue

LIVING WITH UNDIAGNOSED ILLNESS

People receiving a diagnosis of serious illness will often comment that they find it a relief to at least know what is wrong. Knowing, even when the news isn't good, is less traumatic than not knowing.

Living with undiagnosed symptoms for so long created an assortment of paradoxes and double binds. I have talked to many others in similar predicaments and have learned that I wasn't alone in many of the feelings I experienced through my ordeal. Eventually I learned that many diseases aside from Lyme, such as MS, SLE, rheumatic conditions and neurological disorders, often are not easily diagnosed in the early stages. They may not show up on tests and often present vague or overlapping signs.

Undiagnosed conditions create a dilemma for all involved including the patient, the patient's family and the physician.

I found, as time went on, that I became increasingly hesitant to let out all the stops and tell the full story of my illness for fear it wouldn't be believable. At the same time I feared if I didn't share everything, I might omit an important clue that could open the door to eventual diagnosis.

I felt I had to keep tight control over my feelings to avoid being further labeled as hypochondriac, neurotic, hysterical. I found myself trying to be stoic, to "look good" in order to get help.

I spent a great deal of time questioning my own reactions to the signals I was recieving from my own body. There were times I pushed myself and tried to hide or deny disabilities. I blamed myself and felt guilty for what I couldn't do.

When I consulted doctors who suggested that I was

bringing on my condition myself, my clinic visits became avenues to more self-doubt and shattered hopes rather than sources of help.

I have talked to people who have given up and refused to go back to their doctors, fearing they will only be discounted, accused and rejected further.

When I focused my attention on trying to solve my own riddle, some labeled me as obsessing or "dwelling on my symptoms." I wanted to accept my condition and move on, but without a diagnosis or prognosis I found it extremely difficult to do. I perceived many doctors misinterpreting a desire to have answers as a compulsion to be sick. When a person lives with a chronic illness for which there is no explanation, it's extremely difficult not to dwell on the sickness. They usually don't allow themselves to go through the natural grieving process. Fear, anger, and sorrow are pathways to eventual acceptance of any loss. When a person doesn't know what they are grieving for, it's difficult to move beyond the fear.

I realize that it's not always possible for physicians to diagnosis problems and that psychological aspects need to be considered. However, a little tact and compassion on the part of the physician can go a long way in boosting morale and helping the undiagnosed patient to cope.

Prior to my diagnosis, it helped me to talk to others with undiagnosed conditions, to swap information with those who could understand the frustrations I was dealing with, and to offer in turn my consolation and emphathy.

Jean and I have talked about the possibility of forming a support group for persons in the midst of living with undiagnosed illnesses. If you think this would be helpful, please drop us a note and we'll see what we can do. Send

Epilogue

comments to Linda Hanner, 9050 Co. Rd. 11, Maple Plain, MN 55359.

For those living with long-term chronic illness, the following organization can refer you to a group specific to your condition: MINNESOTA MUTUAL HELP RESOURCE CENTER, c/o Wilder Foundation, 919 Lafond Avenue, St. Paul, MN 55104.

DEPRESSION

Through my own experiences and through other resources I have come to realize that depression, in addition to being a disease condition in itself, can occur as a component of illness or as a result of life-events. It may result from a biochemical imbalance or as a side effect of medication. Most people describe feeling depressed at some point during their lives. Depression comes in many different degrees. Sometimes it is manageable, at other times it is severe and some kind of outside help is needed.

Having experienced severe suicidal depression, I feel I am more able to empathize with people who have mental or emotional problems. Often it is difficult to know how to deal with those who are depressed. It is easy to become impatient with them, especially when they don't seem to respond to advice and help that is being offered.

The following suggestions may be of some help:
• Avoid empty phrases such as "I know you'll be fine." A severely depressed person cannot see the positive side of anything.
• Understand that the depressed person might find it extremely difficult to face people, even close friends and

relatives. They may feel forced to act like everything is okay when they can't believe it ever will be.

• Avoid preaching, judging, or accusing.

• Recognize that depression may have nothing to do with the amount of faith a person does or doesn't have. The Bible is filled with stories of faith-filled people who went through depressions and felt rejected or abandoned by God at some point. Even Jesus, as He hung on the cross, questioned why God had abandoned him.

• Bible reading and prayer in the midst of depression may be difficult and may even make the depressed person feel worse than they already do. I believe the prayers of others were extremely important, and I am grateful that I can once again draw comfort from scripture and my own communications with God.

• If the depressed person is willing to talk, try to listen with empathy. Be as accepting, understanding, and non-judgmental as possible. I don't believe that anyone wants to be depressed.

• Encourage the despairing person to seek help through professional resources. However, realize it may take several attempts before a comfortable match between patient and counselor can be found.

• Suicidal people are people whose depression has become so severe they have lost ability to recognize that their terrible feelings will pass with time. They have lost the ability to comprehend anything beyond their own sense of hopelessness. Sometimes medications are helpful, sometimes they make the situation worse. People who are on anti-depressants and tranquilizers should be monitored carefully.

Epilogue

Some books that were helpful to me were:
*Depression: Finding Hope and Meaning in Life's Darkest
Shadow*, by Don Baker. Multnomah Press, Portland,
OR. 1983.

Why Christians Break Down, by William A. Miller.
Augsburg Fortress, Minneapolis, MN. 1973.

DEALING WITH THE MEDICAL PROFESSION

At the onset of my illness I believed that as the patient I
could and should turn over responsibility for my condition
to the doctors, the higher authorities, those with the license
to practice medicine. Now, I feel that the patient and doctor
can and should work together as a team when it comes to
diagnosis and treatment of medical conditions.

While I respect the number of years doctors spend in
rigorous training, I recognize their humanness. During my
years of searching for answers I encountered nearly thirty
doctors. In that time, seldom did two doctors come to the
same conclusion regarding any aspect of my illness. I have
come to believe that the majority of doctors' conclusions are
based on educated guesses, which are often wrong. Their
judgment is subject not only to human error but to inconsis-
tent scientific opinions as well. Medical tests, even when
performed correctly and accurately, have their own rates of
error. Every patient reacts differently to medications, and
often side effects of medications are more difficult to
tolerate than the symptoms they are intended to correct.

Through my own experience I have learned to take
responsibility for communicating my needs, asking about

LYME DISEASE: My Search for a Diagnosis

options, seeking additional opinions and asking for sources of information.

I would encourage patients, especially those who have complex medical cases, to request copies of medical records. Inaccurate and incomplete records, when passed on to other doctors, can cause misunderstanding, faulty conclusions and hinder diagnosis. In my own situation, I allowed my confidence to become eroded by the mental health labels affixed to me by a doctor who later admitted he had applied them inaccurately without good supporting data. Information regarding my medical history and test results were not always completely or accurately recorded before being passed to other clinics. According to several medical professional associations, such as the Minnesota Association of Health Care Facilities, patients do have the right to request copies of medical records.

In spite of the shortcomings of some who were involved in my health care over the past years, I retain a high opinion of the medical profession in general, but feel there is much room for improvement in doctor-patient relationships.

My purpose in writing my story is not to turn people against the medical profession. And I don't wish to encourage people to react by taking everything into their own hands and discounting their doctor's advice. However, I would like to encourage people to trust their own instincts and beliefs and to seek respectful and competent care.

I discovered some exceptional doctors. These doctors stood out not because of a greater amount of knowledge, but because of their ability to recognize and respond to the emotional needs of their patients as well as the physical. The following is a list of qualities I recognized in the doctors who were most helpful to me in dealing with my own predicament:

• Expressed empathy and compassion through simple phrases, such as "I know that this must be very difficult for you to deal with."
• Encouraged calls between visits if questions or concerns arose. Maybe some doctors are afraid of being bombarded with calls if they make this suggestion. Although I seldom called between appointments, knowing I had permission to do so felt reassuring and reduced my anxiety level greatly.
• Encouraged my involvement in decision making and seemed to welcome my own suggestions and comments in regard to treatments.
• Took time to explain risks, possible negative side effects of drugs, and answer questions.
• Seemed to feel comfortable in saying "I don't know," and acknowledging the limits of their professsion or their own experience.
• Showed interest in how other members of the family were dealing with my illness and were interested in my spouse's input.
• Didn't balk at referring me to other doctors or seeking other opinions when the answers weren't clear.

SPIRITUAL UNDERSTANDINGS

Before the illness, I believed that as a Christian I needed to strive to be super human, to be a perfect role model for others. I now am more accepting of my own shortcomings and imperfections and I believe that God can work through me in spite of them. God created me; I have committed my life to Him and I don't need to earn His love. Imperfection doesn't mean failure.

I believed that as a Christian I had to be stoic and mask

feelings such as anger and discouragement. Now I believe that God gave me feelings and accepts all of them in me. Even Jesus became angry, discouraged, and wept. When I express my feelings appropriately, instead of denying them, they become positive emotions. I believe in forgiving others, but it is also okay to express my anger when I believe I have been wronged. If I believe I am being discounted or treated disrespectfully or inappropriately, I can confront the situation.

I believed that as a Christain I had to be strong. Now, I know that at times I will be strong and at times I will be weak. Either is okay. God can bring strength from my weakness.

I believed that I needed to have answers. Now I believe that I will have the answers that I need in God's perfect time.

I believed that I had to be a giver and not a receiver. I hated having people do things for me. I felt guilty. Now I believe that receiving can be a way of giving. I understand that others may need to show their love by offering help. Yet at times I can decide to refuse help tactfully without rejecting the giver. I may never be able to repay specifically the helper of the moment, but I am committed to helping others whenever I can.

I believed that I must reject myself in order to honor God. I now love and believe in God and myself. God exists both within me and apart from me. I don't need to apologize for my feelings, symptoms, thoughts, wishes, dreams or needs. It's okay to be human!

Before, I relied on other people's faith in my faith. Now I feel I can rely on the love and respect I've learned to have for myself. I can't assure that others will love me or won't abandon me, but I can survive with God's love and I believe in my own self-worth.

Some things I am able to change; others I am not. The challenge is to discern between the two. The serenity prayer of the twelve-step program composed by Reinhold Niebuhr isn't always easy to put into practice, but it's worth striving for:

> *God, grant me the serenity*
> *To accept the things I cannot change*
> *Courage to change the things I can*
> *And the wisdom to know the difference.*